ERN

HIS BRAIN WON'T

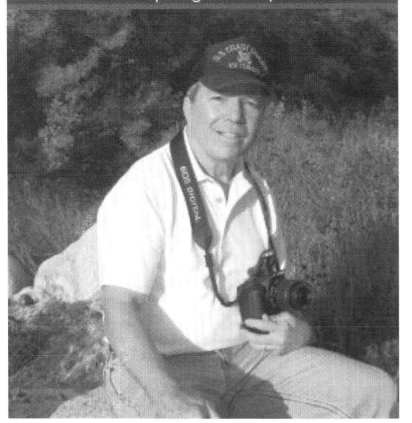

REBOOT

Coping with this rare disease called
"Primary Progressive Aphasia"

His Brain Won't Reboot

Coping with this rare disease called
"Primary Progressive Aphasia"

© 2015 by Ernestina Connolly

Published by:
Ernestina Connolly
erni@verizon.net
www.fcfppa.com

First Printing, 2015

Printed in the United State of America
ISBN: 978-1505352573

Disclaimer

This book is not intended as a substitute for the medical advice of physicians. The reader should regularly consult a physician in matters relating to his/her health and particularly with respect to any symptoms that may require diagnosis or medical attention.

No part of this book may be reproduced or transmitted in any form with the intention of reselling or distributing such copies without written permission from the publisher, except for brief quotations included in a review.

All content and information contained within the book and any related material, service, or product purchased, recommended, or made available is provided "as is" without representations and warranties of any kind, either expressed or implied, including, but not limited to, warranties of merchantability, fitness for a particular purpose, title, or non-infringement. With respect to any third-party products or services described or made available in connection with the book or other materials.

Any warranty provided in connection with such third-party products or services is provided solely by the third-party provider of such products or services and not by the publisher or its owners, sponsors, or agents.

The purchaser and/or user of the book and any related materials assume total responsibility and risk for use of the book and any related products or services. No statement in the book, unless indicated, has been evaluated by the U.S. Food and Drug Administration.

No products mentioned or eluded to are intended to diagnose, treat, cure, or prevent any disease unless authorized by the governing agency at the time of purchase and/or utilization.

Information contained in the book and related materials are intended as an educational aid only.

Information is not intended as medical advice for individual conditions or treatment and is not a substitute for a medical examination, nor does it replace the need for services provided by medical professionals or independent determinations.

A person's individual doctor must determine what is safe and effective for each individual person or patient.

The publisher or its owners, sponsors, or agents do not assume any responsibility or risk for the use of any information contained within the book, or other materials which could contain inaccuracies or errors, and where third parties could make unauthorized additions, deletions, and alterations without the author's knowledge.

Although the author, the publisher and its owners, sponsors, or agents have done their best to ensure full integrity throughout all media, they make no guarantees whatsoever regarding the accuracy, comprehensiveness, and utility of the work.

Table of Contents

Introduction

My name is Ernestina Connolly. I am the fourth to the youngest of eleven children.

In May of 1966 we emigrated from Tijuana, Mexico when I was only four years old.

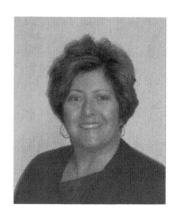

My father worked hard and saved his money so that he could move his family to California.

My uncle and aunts helped my parents obtain green cards so that we could move to California.

I don't remember my early years in Tijuana, but what I do remember is that I fell onto a cactus plant while playing with my sisters in the back yard of our home and my mom had to pull each thorn from my butt.

When we moved to California, my parents, brothers and sisters lived with our grandmother Cecilia in Pasadena, California. I believed we lived in Pasadena for about 4 months. What I do remember about living in Pasadena is that I wanted to go to school to learn English.

Soon after, we moved from Pasadena to Los Angeles, about 20 miles away from our grandmother's home.

My father worked as a welder for a small company in Pasadena, where he earned $3.75 an hour. He worked hard and never called in sick or took a vacation. Then, in September of 1966, with the help of my two oldest sisters, our father was able to purchase a modest 4 bedroom two story home with only one bathroom and an extra shower in the girl's bedroom with a big back yard for all of us kids to play in. My father loved gardening and planted various fruit trees which produced an abundance of fruits for us children to pick during the summer months.

Soon after I started Kindergarten and was learning how to speak English and then in 1967, my brother Rene was born.

I have to say that I had the best childhood any child could have. My mother was a stay at home mom. She was 5'1" with light brown eyes, 120 lbs., and had long dark brown hair. She would make home-made tortillas at least twice a week and was a great cook. When we got home from school, dinner was ready and my brothers and sisters would all eat together.

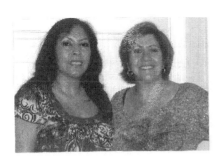

Rose and Erni

As soon as we finished our homework we could play all afternoon until it got dark. The two things I hated most while growing up were having to come in from playing all day outside with my friends and having to take a bath.

Life was so simple then, no internet, no cellphones, no iPads, and definitely no worries, at least not until I became a teenager, then everything changed, but that's another story.

I met my two best friends who are still in my life today, Rachel and Rose. A little later I'll tell you more about them and what a big part of my life they were and still are.

Why I'm writing this book

I'm not a professional writer or a medical researcher, but I'm writing this book to educate the public about the medical condition called Primary Progressive Aphasia ("PPA") and what we can do to encourage more research to find a cure.

This book is for anyone who's experiencing the frustration and anxiety of the disease and what Dan, aka "Sweetiepie" and I went through before we found out about this rare condition.

I have never written a book but my whole experience about how PPA affected Dan and what we went through changed our lives forever.

I want everyone to know about this condition so that I can help others deal with the frustration and emotional rollercoaster you go through when someone you love is diagnosed with PPA.

It includes information about what age group can get it, what signs to look for when you think your loved one has it, what you can do to help your loved one with this condition, the resources available to you, how it affected our lives, and what I did to overcome the frustration that came with knowing my husband, best friend, and lover has Aphasia.

My qualifications for writing this book are simple–I've been there, done that, lived through it; and I still am! I have firsthand experience in dealing with a loved one (my husband Dan) who developed and lives with Primary Progressive Aphasia and what I did to help better our lives in dealing with this condition.

My goal is to educate the public about PPA and get the funds needed for more medical research in finding a cure for this devastating condition.

Here's hoping my experiences will help you and your family to understand and cope.

Dedication

I want to dedicate this book to my Sweetiepie, because without you, my life is not complete.

To my childhood friend Rachel Rodriguez, who came back into my life and who assisted me in writing this book.

To my dear friend Marichelle Maloney, and her family, for always being there for me and Dan and for all your love and support.

To my niece Nicki Hernandez, for your positive encouragement, and for believing Dan was not doing all those things on purpose and that he loves me.

To my sister Margaret, for her love and support and for continued help with Dan.

To all my family and friends, who supported me and helped me with Dan. I couldn't have done it without you.

To my brother-in-law Mike Connolly, who was able to sell all of Dan's motorcycles (9 to be exact) and get them out of my garage and for your continued love and support. I know Dan is very appreciative for all that you do for us, especially the close bond you two have developed and the love you have for one another.

To Helena Chui, M.D., for diagnosing Dan's medical condition and guiding me through this process, and to her staff for all their hard work and dedication.

To Mike Rounds, author, for believing in me, and for giving me the confidence to write this book. It's true, what you said to me when I decided to write this book. "When you are passionate about something and know what you are talking about, the words just seem to flow." For your encouragement and countless hours of editing and re-editing. And, just when I said it was the last edit, you were patient with me when I added more to the book.

To my amazing dad, Eusebio Dominguez, who taught me so much. I will forever be grateful. He passed away on December 20, 2014. I love you and miss you. You will forever remain in my heart.

Chapter 1

The Whole Story – the Condensed Version

Keep reading–it'll get more interesting–I promise☺)

This is a story about me, Ernestina (Erni), my husband, Dan, my family and friends, and a little known medical condition called Primary Progressive Aphasia or "PPA" which is a rare, and often misdiagnosed medical condition.

PPA causes a whole host of strange and misunderstood problems and not just for the person who has it, but for the family, friends, and people who have to interact with that person.

After reading more about PPA and all the signs associated with this condition, I can now look back and see things more clearly and remember all the things that Dan would or wouldn't do that changed his whole personality which caused me to be frustrated and angry with him.

I'm sure it was as frustrating for Dan as it was for me.

It first began with Dan not being sociable with my family and friends. Just saying hello or goodbye was an issue.

As a result, I would constantly argue with him about his social etiquette.

Then came his lack of social interaction with family and friends. I felt like he was jealous that I was spending time with our friends and family and that he wanted me all to himself. This wasn't the person I met just five years prior.

He began to come home late from work and would not call to tell me he was working late. I would make dinner and wait for him to arrive.

I would call him and ask why he didn't call to tell me he would be home late or would not be having dinner with me. This infuriated me. He would just say that he was sorry and that he had to take care of a problem at work.

This was all happening to the point that I thought maybe he was having an affair, because our sex life was non-existent as well.

He wouldn't have sex with me anymore and would often say he was too tired or that we could have fun over the weekend.

The weekend would come and go and Dan would find some excuse why he didn't want to have sex with me. What man turns down sex from his wife?

I have always been sexually active and for me not having sex was driving me crazy. I was frustrated to the point that I wanted to have an affair just for the intimacy, which I was not getting at home.

At one point, I called three of my prior lovers and asked if they would have sex with me because my husband was not giving mc what I wanted. To my surprise, 1 of the 3 said no.

The one I thought would definitely say yes turned me down. He was now married and I thought because he really loved me and we had remained friends that he would say yes.

I was disappointed that he said no, but I understood and respected him for that.

And no, I didn't have sex with the other two, but I was very close to doing so.

I contacted my therapist and told him what I was contemplating, we talked and somehow I was able to calm down and all my anxiety and frustrations went away.

Chapter 2

Before the Diagnosis

Prior to Dan being diagnosed with Primary Progressive Aphasia, he was passionate about his job and knew all there is to know about computers. He worked for large engineering firm in Los Angeles, California.

Dan is a numbers man; he can remember any number or password you give him.

I don't know how he remembers numbers, but he did, and still does. While working at the engineering firm, he managed three offices in Southern California, one office in San Diego and one office in Seattle, Washington.

Dan could fix anything and if he didn't know how to do fix something, he would learn how to do it.

He would often spend hours at home testing programs and finding out how to clone them. This was to enable his office to see the same thing the other offices were doing so as to not duplicate the same work.

Each person working on a project could see what was going on in another office or state without duplicating or shutting down the system because of too many users.

Dan was the go-to person everyone went to get their computers fixed, whether it was at the office or outside of the office.

Many people would say that Dan has a radio voice. He is well spoken, and has a calming voice when explaining to you what is going on with your computer.

Dan could walk you through the process, over the phone, about how to install a program or find a file, or just about anything you need. That's how knowledgeable he was. He was so smart and I would tell him how smart I thought he was every chance I had. He could build anything and fix anything that needed to be fixed.

He was so talented and so smart that I believe I fell in love with him because of his intelligence and because he was so down to earth. He would help anyone that needed help and would always think of others before himself. In my eyes, he was a genius and still is.

Dan's other passion was in motorcycles. He enjoyed collecting vintage motorcycles and restoring them. He had 5 Triumph, 2 Norton, and 2 Harley Davidson motorcycles. Dan liked his 2002 red and silver Harley Davidson Springer the best, which we would ride often.

Dan enjoyed listening to live music and loved turning the music up loud in the house. He especially liked playing music for others. He has a 300,000+ collection of music and would play for you almost any music you wanted to hear.

Due to his medical condition, Dan can no longer enjoy doing the things he loves to do, like work on computers and help others. He can no longer drive a car, or ride his Harley Davidson motorcycle (which he loved to ride every chance he could). In fact, we had to sell all of his motorcycles because he no longer has the stimulation or passion he once had in working on the motorcycles.

It was Dan's decision to sell the motorcycles and with his brother Mike's help, we were able to sell all the motorcycles.

Before we sold Dan's 2002 Harley Davidson Springer, he had a chance to take it for one last ride. Dan knew he was not allowed to drive, but I took the chance and allowed him to ride the motorcycle from our home in Glendora to his brother's home 55 miles away. I was nervous about Dan driving the motorcycle because his driver's license had just been taken from him 3 months earlier. Dan had a big smile on his face when I told him he could ride his bike to his brother's home.

It was a sunny Saturday morning and the temperature outside was about 73 degrees. I watched Dan get on his bike and I said a prayer and followed him in the car as he drove down the street and onto the freeway to his brother's home. I got my video camera, placed it on the dashboard of our car and video-taped Dan riding his motorcycle for the last time.

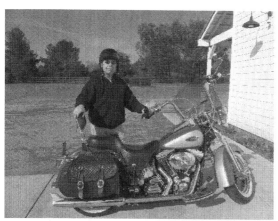

Dan's last ride

Because Dan was an excellent

8

rider I was not worried about him riding the bike, I was more worried about someone running into him than anything else.

When we made it to Dan's brother's house, Dan made a gesture that it was cold riding the bike. I said, I know, you did perfect. Dan smiled at me and said, "I did everything perfect."

When it was time to sell the Harley Davidson Springer Dan was not sad because he knew that the person who bought it would enjoy riding it as much as he did, plus he knew he would be getting a pretty good amount of money for it, which made him happy.

Dan can no longer read and write, understand conversations going on around him or comprehend information given to him.

Dan can no longer enjoy the physical intimacy we once had. In fact, we don't even have a sex life.
Not having a sex life really frustrated me until I found out what was wrong with Dan.

After I found out what was wrong with Dan, our sex life was not that important to me anymore.

What became important is how I can help my husband get better or somehow slow down the process of his condition.

Just knowing there was something wrong with Dan made a big difference our marriage.

You see, before we found out that Dan had Primary Progressive Aphasia, our relationship was headed downhill.

Chapter 3

The Decisions You Make Dictate Your Future

It was Sunday, February 21, 2010; I was in our bedroom in our home in Glendora, California. Dan and I had a huge fight.

We had been to see our CPA 3 weeks prior to get our taxes done and on our drive home, I was talking to Dan about the fact that we were going to get a nice return from the IRS and I asked him what he wanted to do with the money. He didn't respond and just stared out the window. I then said hey, I'm talking to you, why don't you answer me, what's wrong with you, aren't you happy that we are getting a nice return back from the IRS? Dan replied that it was his money because he made more money than I. I was furious that he made that comment and responded, fine take that money and shove it up your ass you asshole, don't talk to me anymore. We drove in silence the entire drive home.

When we got home, I went to my room and told Dan not to talk to me anymore. I was so upset that he said that to me. We never argued about money or the fact that Dan made more money than I. Then I remembered that Dan had once made a comment years earlier that he bought the house with his money and that I didn't contribute towards the down payment and that it was his house. When I thought about that, it infuriated me even more.

That incident started an argument again and I specifically remember this date because all I wanted to do was kill myself.

I was tired of all the arguing and lack of trust in our relationship and the fact that we were not having sex or even communicating with one another. I felt helpless and didn't know where to go or who to turn too.

I had stopped taking my anti-depressant medication at that time and my depression had returned. Dan was in the other bedroom and all I could think of was that he would find me dead and would regret how he treated me.

I was so depressed and upset that I got a gun that Dan had in the bottom drawer of his dresser, kneeled on our bed, put the gun up to my head, and attempted to pull the trigger. Somehow, I couldn't get the gun to go off, tears were running down my face and all I wanted to do is die.

The gun was an antique which had belonged to Dan's father or grandfather. All I wanted was to get out of this relationship and the only way I was going to do it was by shooting myself.

I felt like my husband was no longer the person I fell in love with and married 4 years prior. We didn't talk anymore, have dinner together because he was always working late, and our intimacy deteriorated and we no longer even slept in the same bed.

All I could think of is why I didn't just leave when I filed for divorce in October of 2007, why was I still here, because I couldn't continue to live this way.

When the gun didn't go off, I didn't know what else to do but to cry myself to sleep. I am so grateful the gun hadn't gone off; otherwise, I wouldn't be here to tell my story and Dan's story about his medical condition.

Many people don't realize that the decisions you make, whether big or small, dictate your future and the future of your entire family.

My decision to kill myself would have been a BIG mistake, because as you continue to read about our triumphs and tribulations, you will see that there is a higher power out there keeping us from making what could be the biggest mistake of our lives.

For those of you who have never experienced severe depression, it's hard to explain what you are feeling and what you are going through, let alone admit to your family that you are depressed. You don't want your family to know that you are depressed for fear they will worry about you. In my case, I was ashamed that I was on anti-depressants for my depression and didn't want my family to know. When you are severely depressed and in a state of mind of destruction, you are not thinking rationally, you're not thinking about your family and friends, or how devastating it will be to them that you took your life and that there was nothing they could do to help you. All you are thinking about in that moment in time is how much pain you are going through and you want the pain to go away. I'm not sure if anyone knew how depressed I really was and the extent I went through to stop the pain.

14

I can't even image what Dan's life would have been like had I continued to go through with the divorce proceedings in 2007 or succeeded in killing myself.
Would Dan have gone to the doctor to see what was wrong with him? Would his family understand what he was going through, or would they think he was just depressed because of another failed marriage? Would he have lost his job eventually because he would be unable to perform the duties of his job?

Or would he have gone into a severe depression or even worse, killed himself? What a tragedy that would have been.

Because Dan's medical condition is often misdiagnosed, many men don't understand what's going on and won't go see a doctor or even talk to a loved one or a family member about what they are going through.

I say many men, because women tend to see a doctor more often than men when they feel something is not right with them. I can only tell you from my experience with Dan, that staying with him and getting him the medical attention he needed was the best thing I could have done for Dan and for our marriage.
Could there be others with Primary Progressive Aphasia going through what Dan went through who may not be aware of this condition?

Ernestina Connolly

Chapter 4

Our Lives Before The Diagnosis (05/2007-05/2011)

Our lives before finding out that my husband had Primary Progressive Aphasia were rollercoasters.

I'm sure Dan was as frustrated as I was because he didn't understand what was going on as well.

Dan took pride in his work, whether it be fixing a computer, replacing a window in our home, changing the oil in his car, or building a closet. It had to be done right and perfect.

I'm sure he was having difficulty understanding why certain things which had come easy for him were now taking longer to do.

He didn't know how to explain what was happening to him or maybe he was afraid to tell me that he was forgetting things because he was getting older. Then he had me yelling at him all the time because he would come home late every night and not call. In addition, he was less interested in our sex life. He probably thought; *why is this person whom I married bashing me every chance she gets?*

His attitude was: I work hard to provide for her and all she thinks about is sex and why I'm not home on time.

It wasn't just the sex and coming home late, it was that we were not communicating.

Every time I would ask Dan to do something for me or to get ready by a certain time because we were going somewhere, Dan would say ok.

18

But then when it was time to go or do something Dan would either not do it, or would not be ready to go when I got home.

This behavior would often start an argument with me yelling at him as to why he did not do what I asked him to do, or why was he not ready to go when I got home. His reply every time would be, okay, I'll do it, or, give me two seconds.

For example, taking out the trash on Sunday evening or Monday morning was an issue.

If I didn't do it, the trash would not get picked up.

He would work on a project inside the house and get sanding dust everywhere and would not clean it up. I would clean it up and then would tell him to make sure he puts up plastic around the door ways to ensure the dust remains in one room and he would say okay. Then, when I would get home, dust would be everywhere again and he would have no clue why I was so upset.

He also began to leave tools out and not put them away in their proper place, which infuriated me, because I would often trip over them. He would also leave sharp objects out in the back yard where the dogs could get hurt. I again would remind him time and time again to put the tools away and clean up after his mess. And again, this type of behavior would start an argument. I would say, how many time do I have to tell you to pick up after yourself, I'm tired of

19

cleaning up after your mess. Again, he would say, okay, I'll do it.

Dan's social skills were diminishing as well. He would not say hello to my friends or family when they would talk to him, and that would get me all worked up.

I would ask him; *why are you not socializing with my friends and family, what is wrong with you, why did I bring you,* or I would simply say, *you should have just stayed home.*

Dan would only communicate with family or friends if the topic of conversation was about computers or motorcycles. He could talk your ears off if the subject came up about computers or motorcycles. He knew everything there was to know about computers and motorcycles and felt comfortable talking to anyone who would listen to him. But when it came to other topics of conversation, Dan would only nod his head or occasionally say okay to what you were talking about.

This type of behavior went on for years and then I thought maybe he had a hearing problem, so I took him to get his hearing checked.

When we found out that it was not his hearing, I wondered what it could be because he's just not the man I married anymore.

Do spouses actually change after you get married?

All I could think of was a way to get out of this relationship because I was not happy anymore and I didn't want to be with someone who wasn't willing to make this marriage work.

Then the question hit me; where would I go? I didn't make enough money to stay in our home.

Dan was not going to leave and I was not ready to get a place of my own, and what about our dogs?

I couldn't leave them with Dan because he would forget to feed them or make sure they had water.

I couldn't let that happen. What was I to do?

I tried to make our marriage work but it was like a broken record. The same issues and problems were going on every week and the weeks turned into months and before you knew it, the months turned into years.

Then when you have had enough and cannot take it anymore, you make decisions that you think are the best at the time, or make irrational decisions that could ruin your life and those of your entire family.

My decision to get the help for myself and to seek medical attention for my husband was the best thing that I could have done to save our marriage.

Ernestina Connolly

Chapter 5

About Me

About me

One of the things that we all need to remember about debilitating disease is that it is not about the disease but the people that are affected.

Since PPA affected Dan and me, it's good for you to know who we were and who we now are as a result of the disease.

My career

My first job was that of an order clerk for Jack-in-the-Box. I hated that job, the customers were rude and I had to be nice to them. What I hated most was saying "Welcome to Jack-in-the-Box, how may, I help you." You either have that talent or not, and I didn't have it.

After that short-lived job, I worked a summer job at the warehouse department store Broadway, which was okay, but I knew I didn't want to do that line of work the rest of my life. I then worked for a precision products company answering phones, which I didn't like either. I think I got fired from that job after 3 months. After those few jobs, I decided to stay in college for as long as I could.

While in college I took a business law class and that's how I got into the field of law and became a Legal Secretary. I have over 25 years' experience in family law and currently work for a civil litigation law firm.

Being in the legal field also helped me to understand the law and know what our rights are. I am very fortunate to have the knowledge and ability to research what is available for Dan and how to fill out the correct forms and applications so that Dan can get all the benefits he is entitled to through our government system.

My interests

I love animals, music, especially the blues, I love to travel and see how the other half of the world lives. I enjoy taking photos of people, places and animals, and nature. I love to dance, help others and make others happy.

I used to enjoy reading novels and autobiographies and all of John Grisham and Patricia Cornwell books, until I got married and now don't have time to read anymore.

All my free time is spent with my Sweetiepie, doing things together and making his life simple and happy. I wish I had more time to spend with Dan, but I have to work to help support us financially. After working all day, being on the computer at work and coming home and paying attention to Dan, I'm simply out of time and energy.

Attitude about family and children

I love my large family of over 80 nieces, nephews and cousins, especially children, so long as they do not belong to me.
You see, working in the legal field for most of my adult life has dissuaded me from having children. Although

my friend Rachel would tell you that I always said at a young age that I would never have children.

Working in the field of family law, you see and hear all that goes on in a relationship. First you fall in love, have a lavish wedding and then come the children.

There is no book that can tell you how to make your marriage last forever without problems or challenges, because no matter how happy you are in a relationship, there are always ups and downs, that's just part of life.

But how you deal with it is what makes a relationship work. I know from firsthand experience that you really don't know an individual until you have lived with them, and that's the truth.

The first two years of a marriage are called the honeymoon stage.

After you've passed the honeymoon stage, it's called the seven-year itch, which means you've either grown apart because you got married too young or didn't get a chance to experience life and now feel that you need something new.

Then there are the spouses that are workaholics and never have time to spend with you, the ones that cheat, are physically or verbally abusive, become addicted to drugs, alcohol, porn, etc. and then comes the divorce.
The man or woman you married becomes this monster and all you want to do is hurt them for becoming this

person you never knew. The love you once had becomes hatred and all you want to do is destroy the other person.

If you have children, they are the ones who are most affected, but spouses don't care about what the divorce is doing to the children because all they want to do is get even with the other spouse for breaking up the marriage.

Then you spend all your hard earned money on attorney's fees, arguing who will get the four sets of Waterford Crystal champagne glasses you got as a wedding present, or argue about keeping the other party's bowling ball or wedding dress just to see the other party upset.

I could write a book about all the things parties fight over that run up attorney's fees, but that's another story.

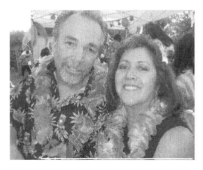

Dan and Erni

After seeing this happen year after year, I said I would never get married or have children.

I stuck with my promise of never having children, but I finally did decide to get married at the age of 45 to my best friend and soul-mate which you will learn more about in this book.

27

Ernestina Connolly

Chapter 6

How We First Met

I first met my Sweetiepie in 1999, while working for a prestigious family law firm in Santa Monica, California. Dan was an IT person for a local computer software and technical support company in Santa Monica.

Dan was the most knowledgeable of his co-workers and he was assigned to assess our computer system in preparation for Y2K which was soon approaching.

I didn't take much interest in Dan in the beginning. However, as soon as I found out that Dan was the person to call when things didn't get done right, I requested that only Dan fix our computer problems and update our software.

Dan was so much in demand that sometimes it would take 2 or 3 weeks to get him to come to our office to fix whatever was wrong. One day, Dan showed up dressed in a pair of Dockers beige pants and a black crew neck shirt. The only thing that I noticed at the time was Dan's cute little buttocks. I didn't find Dan attractive in the beginning.

Dan was 5'8" and weighed 163 lbs. He had dark brown shoulder length hair with some gray starting to come in, and wore bifocal eye glasses. He had a noticeable mole on his right cheek. Not my typical guy, but Dan was so personable and easy to talk to and extremely knowledgeable in computer software and hardware that I kept my eye on him.

In early 2002, Dan asked me out a couple of times but each time I told him I had plans. I really did have plans, but had I found Dan to be more attractive, I would have cancelled my plans.

Soon Dan was at our office again working on our computers and to my surprise, on October 25, 2002, Dan asked me out again. Dan had indicated that he and his partner Bill had their own business, selling Bonneville motorcycle parts and were going to be at Hansen Dam, in the Valley, for a Harley Davidson Motorcycle show. He asked if I would come and see their event booth.

This time I said yes, and told him I would meet him there in the mid afternoon as soon as I was done with my golf game.

I got to Hansen Dam around 2:30 p.m. and was looking for Dan's booth. I saw Dan from a distance and I wasn't sure if it was him because the person I was looking at had short hair and was not wearing eye glasses.

To my surprise, when I got closer, it was Dan. He looked so much better with short hair and no eye glasses. He was glad to see me and gave me a big hug.

It was nice spending time with Dan and getting to know him outside of a work setting. We walked around and had a chance to view the Harley Davidson motorcycles that were on display. Some were entered in a contest for the best looking bike. Dan was

31

surprised that I guessed which motorcycles would be the top three.

The only reason I knew about Harley Davidson motorcycles was because one of my old boyfriends had a Harley Davidson and we would often go to bike shows.

We ended our evening about 6 p.m. and Dan asked what I was doing on November 10th. I told him I didn't know, that I would check my calendar, and get back with him next week.

Dan called me the following week and asked if I wanted to join him in the Harley Davidson Love Ride which would take place on November 10th in Glendale, California. Dan said there would be hundreds of Harley Davidson motorcycles and that it was a big event.

To make a long story short, I went to the Love Ride with Dan and we had the best time. We had a chance to really talk and get to know one another more. We enjoyed the wonderful music, great food and soon started dating.

I'm glad that Dan didn't give up and continued to pursue me and that I finally said yes! After the Love Ride, Dan and I became inseparable and within 6 months we moved in together. As you read more about Dan's medical condition and our story, you will find that things happen for a reason in life and that meeting Dan was meant to be, otherwise, he wouldn't

have me to take care of him and I wouldn't have him to
love.

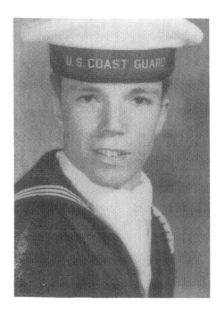

Dan US Coast Guard 1973

Ernestina Connolly

Chapter 7

Dan's background and Career

Dan enlisted in the U.S. Coast Guard in 1973 because he did not want to get drafted to Vietnam. He was stationed at Wake Island for 2 years and then in 1974 he was transferred to San Diego.

I really don't know too much about Dan's early years in the Coast Guard but what I do know, from what his cousin Eric has told me, is that Dan was responsible for all the incoming and outgoing goods and services as well as guarding the prisoners and the illegal drugs that were seized.

On one occasion, while Dan and his crewmen were guarding the marijuana, they decided to try it.

They were all having fun smoking, drinking, dancing and getting friendly with the women prisoners. The next thing you know, they had let a few of the women prisoners out to join them in their festivities.

They were all having a wonderful time when suddenly, a Sergeant smelled the Marijuana and proceeded to follow the smell which led him to the young men.

Needless to say, they were all caught in compromising positions. After that incident, Dan and the other young men who took part in the celebration were transferred. Dan was transferred to San Diego to finish his duty.

Dan had many jobs after he returned from the military. He worked as a car salesman, a carpenter, sold paint, electronic equipment and even worked at his father's toy soldier store. By 1994, Dan found his calling in computers.

Because of Dan's photographic memory, he remembers everything especially numbers and anything that has to do with computers. He is familiar with all the ins-n-outs so much so that he could almost do it blindfolded.

Dan was able to help you with your computer, while driving, and walk you through things step by step and tell you where to move the cursor within the computer to get your computer working again.

Dan taught himself at an early age how to fix things. He would take the radio and speakers apart and put them back together again. He would take his bicycle apart and put it back together again. He loved the challenge of taking things apart and putting them back together again without an instruction manual.

One time at the age of 13, Dan's mother told me that he took the dryer apart because it was not working and was able to get the dryer working again. She believed one of the wires was loose and Dan tightened it and put everything back and before you knew it, the dryer was working again.

Dan would often spend hours at work or at home learning all there is to know about computers and the various programs. He could take a computer apart and put it back together again and make it work faster and better than it did before.

Interests

Dan's love for motorcycles began at the age of 12, when his father bought him his first dirt bike. He was a natural and even taught himself how to fix the bike, often taking bikes apart and putting them back together.

As he got older, his interest in motorcycles expanded and before he knew it, he had nine motorcycles in the garage. But the motorcycle he loved best was his 2002 Harley Davidson Springer.

Dan loves animals and music, especially the blues, including music from the 40s, 50s, 60s, 70s, and 80s.

He also enjoyed taking pictures at an early age. I think he got that from his aunt who loved taking pictures. To this date, he still loves taking pictures and has over 50 varieties of cameras.

I think that's what we have most in common, our love of taking pictures, enjoying the same kind of music, and our love for animals (of which we have three; two cocker spaniels, Springer and Sportster, and a poodle named ChuChu).

Attitude about family and children

Dan comes from a very small family. Dan's grandfather, Bobby Connolly, had four children, Bill (Dan's father), Madelyn, Bootsy and Robert. Madelyn had two children, Robert had one child and Bootsy had none. Bobby Connolly died before Dan and his brother Mike were born so Dan didn't get to know his grandfather. Bobby Connolly was in the movie business. He was both a choreographer and a director. He created the dances for around 25 movies, mainly in the 1930s, the best known today being *Flirtation Walk* (1934) and *The Wizard of Oz* (1939).

Dan didn't know his grandmother (from his mother's side) either, she too died soon after Dan and his brother Mike were born.

Dan's father Bill worked for Lockheed Aircraft and because of his job, they moved around a lot. His father was an engineer and in 1968 designed and help build the Lunar Vehicle chemically expanded wheels that NASA used to go to the Moon.

Dan was a shy kid and because Dan and his family moved around a lot, Dan didn't have many close friends while growing up. Dan was in the Cub Scouts and then became an Eagle Scout, which he loved being a part of. He also loved playing the trumpet, which he was very good at.

By the time Dan was a teenager, his parents had moved 7 times. His family finally settled in Burbank, California, where Dan attended Burbank High School.

Dan was very close to his mother, Rosanna, who was a stay-at-home mom. Then, in 1972, Dan's world turned upside down when his parents divorced.

His father was married four times, his aunt was married four times, and his grandfather was married twice.

I believe Dan likes being married, because prior to marrying me (his fourth wife), he was married three times, or maybe it's a Connolly family thing.

When Dan returned from the U.S. Coast Guard in 1974, he married his first wife and divorced a year later.

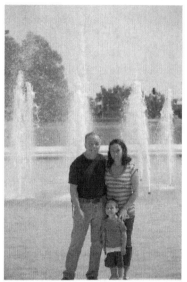

Then he met his second wife in the late 70s and moved to Arizona. They had a daughter named Maureen. Dan was so in love with Maureen's mother, that when she requested he get a vasectomy Dan agreed. Dan believed he would be married to his second wife forever.

Dan with his daughter Maureen & grandson Gino

When Maureen was 3 years old, he and his wife divorced. After the divorce Dan was estranged from his daughter and didn't see too much of her in the early years.

Dan moved back to California in the mid-80s. Later, when his daughter was an adult, she decided to look for her dad and soon they began to have a father/daughter relationship again. Dan was happy that he and his daughter became close once again.

Dan then married his 3rd wife in 1995 and by 1997 there was a breakdown in their marriage and he separated from this wife.

It wasn't until he met me in 1999, and actually started dating me in 2002, that he decided to get a divorce from his 3rd wife. Well actually, I told him he had to get a divorce from his wife if he wanted to continue to date me.

In 2003, Dan filed for divorce, with my help of course, and by October of 2003, he was no longer married.

Dan loves his small family and definitely his extended family too. He may not know all my family members' names, but he sure can show you how to get to their homes.

Ernestina Connolly

Chapter 8

Our Mutual Interests

We both like the out-doors, love taking pictures and going to Coronado Island to relax. We like the same kind of music, especially the blues, and we both are not crazy about rap music. We even like the same kind of foods, taking long walks, and we love to travel. We both enjoyed going for long rides on his Harley Davidson before his license got taken away due to his illness.

We both like the fact that we do not have young children at home and we can walk around the house naked, and go and do whatever we want without having to worry about a babysitter.

We both are honest, faithful, and respect one another. Family is important to us and we spend as much time as possible with our loved ones on the weekends and on holidays. Dan never misses Christmas day at his brother Mike's home.

Our physical intimacy

We both enjoy physical intimacy, and spend lots of time together. We both know what the other person likes and dislikes and respect the other's privacy.

Because of Dan's medical condition, now our physical intimacy primarily involves spending as much time together as possible hugging and kissing, holding hands, and having dinner together every night. We tell one another how much we love each other.

Dan makes it a point every night that we are in bed by 7:00 p.m. to watch his favorite game shows, Jeopardy and Wheel of Fortune. I can't always make it every night because I'm busy doing things around the house, but for the most part, I try and watch the game shows with him at least 3 times a week.

I love to watch Dan have fun watching the contestants win prizes and money. We stare in each other's' eyes and tell one another that we love each other.

On day, while we were watching the game shows, Dan said to me "I did for you in 99 but actually in 2, and I totally love you and it's great."
Which means: He met me in 1999, but we didn't get together until 2002, that he's totally in love with me, and that life is great. That's all I need from him.

The romance in our lives

Before Dan began to develop symptoms of aphasia, we had the perfect life. We would have dinner together every night and talk about our day and what we had planned for the weekend. Dan enjoyed cooking on the BBQ and would often make steak or chicken and sometimes tri-tip and baked potatoes every chance he could.

I'm not a very good cook, as anyone who knows me will tell you (I don't cook). But I would cook dinner for my Sweetiepie and me at least twice a week and would enjoy candlelit dinners together with our Trader Joe's 2-buck Chuck wine, that's until it became very popular and then it was difficult to find at times.

We also played golf and went on short trips on the Harley Davidson to Malibu, Mount Baldy, or we'd just ride around the nearby city to grab a bite to eat.

Dan was an excellent rider and I trusted him with my life. Riding his Harley Davidson always put a smile on Dan's face, which I loved to see. He enjoyed riding with his friends too and always made it a point to be home before it got dark because he didn't want me to worry about him.

He made sure I was always happy and always protected me wherever we went. We never argued and always communicated. We did have our occasional disagreements, but what married couple doesn't? We always respected and trusted one another. Life was great and we enjoyed spending as much time together as we could. Our love life was perfect too. We would make love almost every morning before we left for work and in the middle of the night. Whatever I wanted, Dan made it happen.

We loved going to outdoor concerts and hanging out with our friends and family and we enjoyed taking photos of our family and friends.

We tell each other we love you every morning and before we go to bed. We have nick names for each other; we both call each other "Sweetiepie" and we call each other that everywhere we go, whether it's at the grocery store, shopping, or at family gatherings. We don't care that everyone knows our special name we have for one another.

We try to please the other and do what the other person wants to do, whatever that may be. Before PPA, I would tell Dan "I love you Sweetiepie" and he would say "I love you too." I then would say "how much" and he would say "The Most in The Universe."

Now because of Dan's medical condition, he can no longer say the Most in The Universe, but he replaced that with "I Love You Temporarily Totally," and that works for me.

Dan makes sure I get to work on time, and walks me to the car each morning, gives me a big kiss, and waves good bye. He sometimes calls me at work during the day to say he loves me and to confirm what time I'm coming home so we can have dinner together.

When I get home, he greets me at the door with a big smile and a big hug and a kiss. He often says he wants to order for me. (Which means he wants to take me out to dinner.) After we are done with dinner, Dan sometimes says he wants to order for me for 31. Which means he wants to take me out for ice cream at Baskin Robins.

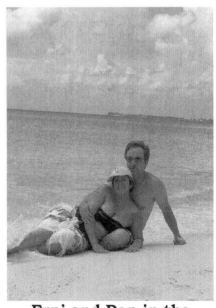

Erni and Dan in the Caymans

47

Sometimes we just lie in bed staring at each other and telling each other "I love you."

Dan is so loving and caring; he would do anything for me. Whatever I want, Dan will try and get it or build it. He always thinks about me when I'm not feeling well. He tells me, "are you still having an error" or "are you normal."

Dan and I love to travel and wherever I want to go, Dan would make it happen, like when we went to the Cayman Islands in 2003. We had the best time ever. We didn't do much, just relaxed on the beach or by the pool and took lots of pictures. We would get up around 9 a.m., have breakfast by the pool, take a long walk on the beach and then relax by the pool. After we had too much sun, we would go to our room and take a long nap, make love, get dressed for dinner, be in bed by 10:00 p.m., and do it again the next day.

The best way to enjoy yourself is to not have an agenda; just get up and do what you feel like doing that day.

Now, because of Dan's condition, it's difficult to go on long trips with him. He is like a child sometimes, doesn't listen, and likes to wander off by himself. He has no sense of fear or danger and often times does

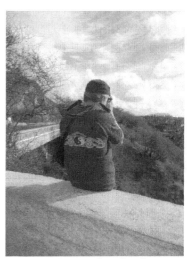

Dan on the ledge

things that could get him killed or seriously hurt.

When we went to Hawaii in 2012, Dan decided to take a picture and went over the wall onto the ledge to get a better camera angle, which made me extremely nervous. I was afraid he would fall down the hill into the ocean.

That trip was also a challenge because Dan was unable to understand everything we were telling him.

On one occasion, Nick, a friend of ours, gave Dan a bag of seeds and told him to give it to the fish. Dan said okay and proceeded to eat the seeds himself. I ran up to Dan and said no, this is for the fish, see, and then I threw some seeds in the water and the fish came up and ate the food. I handed Dan the bag of food for the fish and he proceeded to throw the whole bag of seeds in the pond.

Or in 2011, when we went to Costa Rica, and the raccoon bit his hand.

Now we take small trips to Coronado Island in San Diego, or to Santa Barbara or Carmel. We hold hands while walking on the beach or window shopping. We enjoy a nice dinner and Dan is always near me no matter where we go.

Ernestina Connolly

Chapter 9

Depression

I had been fighting depression for the past year or two before finding out about Dan's condition. I refused to see the doctor because I didn't want to be put on anti-depressant medication and be like all the other thousands of people who were on some type of anti-depressant. I was also ashamed of the possibility of needing medication, and I didn't want my family or friends to know.

I had always been a strong individual or should I say, I was as hard as a rock. I didn't care if anyone said negative things about me. I guess I had the, "I don't give a shit attitude." I said and did whatever I wanted and if you didn't like it, tough. As a young child growing up, my brothers and sisters would always tease me and call me names and say I had a freeway mouth because my teeth were so crooked. (*I showed them, I have straight teeth now*).

When you come from a large family, you learn how to grow a thick skin, because as children, we tend to tease one another and sometimes say bad things to make the other person mad.

When I became a teenager, the Rodriguez brothers would also tease me and say my sister Margaret was prettier than I was, and that my body should be on her face. My body measurements were 34/24/36, just like the song, *Brick House*. I never throught I was pretty enough and that's why the guys never hit on me and would often tease me.

My best friend Rosalie (Rose) would say "don't listen to them, you are much prettier than your sister, they are just mad because you don't pay attention to them like your sister does."

My teenage years were pretty tough and I have to say, I couldn't have made it if it wasn't for my best friend Rose. But again, that's a different story.

In August of 2009, I could no longer handle all that was going on in my life.

I was unhappy in my marriage and unhappy in my job, so I went to see my doctor and told him that I was depressed, not sleeping at night, having trouble concentrating and functioning in my day to day life.

I also told him that driving to and from work was difficult and that I felt like I could not keep my eyes open while driving. I told him that I almost got into an accident because I dosed off while driving.

My doctor had my blood drawn, requested a urine specimen, said that I needed to see a therapist for my depression, and that he would prescribe an anti-depressant.

I told him that I was already seeing a therapist because of all that was going on in my marriage and if he was going to put me on an anti-depressant that I wanted the lowest dose.

A friend of mine was taking the anti-depressant Lexapro® and said she tried several others before going on Lexapro®. Since she had indicated that this anti-depressant worked well for her, I asked my doctor if we could try that medication and see how it worked for me and he said ok.

A week later, I got a call from my doctor with respect to the blood work and he indicated that I had type-2 diabetes and high cholesterol. When I heard the news that I had type 2 diabetes, I was not surprised because a year prior, my doctor had indicated that I was showing signs that I could become diabetic if I did not control my weight and eating habits.

I wasn't obese, just 20 pounds overweight, so he prescribed Metformin for my diabetes and Lisinopril for my cholesterol.

After a month of taking Lexapro, I began to feel better.

My anxiety and frustrations were gone, and so was my sex drive.

I didn't tell anyone except my friend Marichelle and my neighbor Wendy because they were the ones who had suggested I see my doctor and get on some type of anti-depressant. They were the ones who knew the details about the stress I was under, and firsthand knowledge of how angry and frustrated I would get with Dan about not having sex with me and about all the things he was and wasn't doing. Marichelle was always there for me too. I would call her daily and tell her all about my frustrations with Dan and about our non-existent sex life.

Then, in December of 2009, I decided to stop taking my anti-depressant because I was feeling much better.

In February of 2010, my anxiety and frustrations came back and I was once again arguing with Dan about not having sex with me. My depression came back too. I was having a difficult time understanding why I was feeling so depressed all the time.

After getting in another heated argument with Dan, I went over to my neighbor Wendy's house all upset and crying that Dan was not paying attention to me and would not have sex with me. Wendy remembered how upset and frustrated I would get when Dan wouldn't have sex with me, or when he would not do what I asked him to do.

After getting all neurotic worrying and thinking it was the end of the world, Wendy said to me, "Erni, are you taking your medication?" I replied "No, because I was feeling better."

Then she replied, "That's stupid. You were feeling better because you were taking the medication."
Then she asked how long had I been off the medication and I said since December. Her response was to remind me that the reason I was acting neurotic again was the lack of medication and to go home and take the medication.

I said "Okay, so you really think that's what's making me crazy?" and she said "Of course you neurotic sex freak."

We both laughed, she gave me a big hug and said she liked the old Erni and to stay on my meds.

I truly didn't realize that it was the medication that was making me feel better and helping me get through the day without over reacting or feeling depressed. No one should stop taking their medication without the prior consent of their doctor.

I was fortunate to have such great friends who recognized something was not right with me and said I needed help and helped me to understand that sometimes we cannot do it alone.

Chapter 10

Marriage Counseling

I filed for divorce in October of 2007 and served Dan with the divorce papers two weeks later.

When Dan received the divorce papers, he didn't know what to do, and just went to his room when he got home from work. We were already sleeping in separate bedrooms so we didn't really talk anymore.

It wasn't until a week later that Dan finally asked why I was filing for divorce. I told Dan that our marriage wasn't working out and that it was best that we get a divorce. Dan replied "I don't want a divorce, I love you." I replied, "If you love me, then why are you behaving the way you are and not calling me when you are working late and don't do the things I ask you to do? Every time I ask you to do something, you say okay, but then you don't do it. I am tired of arguing with you and its best that we just go our separate ways so that there is no more arguing. I cannot live this way." Dan replied, "What can I do to fix our marriage?"

I told him, "Just leave me alone, I don't want to deal with this anymore, I'm tired of fighting and yelling at you, I can't do this anymore. I'd rather be by myself than to be with someone who doesn't pay attention to me and communicate with me."

Dan replied, "I will do whatever you want me to do, but don't leave me, I don't want a divorce." I then said I needed some time to think about it and to please leave me alone. He said okay.

58

The next couple of weeks Dan was making an effort to come home on time and have dinner with me.   We would have dinner together, but neither of us would say much at dinnertime.   It was strange because we would just sit and eat our dinner and only say one or two words to each other.   Then, Dan would ask if I could come and watch TV with him in his room. I said okay, and we would just lie in bed and watch TV and not talk to one another.

It was now late November and Thanksgiving was approaching.   I asked Dan if he wanted to have Thanksgiving at home and that I would pick up something or if he wanted to go to his mother's house and we could have Thanksgiving with her.

Dan said whatever I wanted to do was okay with him.

I said okay, I will call your mother and see what she is doing and maybe we can have Thanksgiving with her.
We began Marriage Counseling shortly thereafter.   I went to the first three sessions by myself and then asked Dan to come along.   During our first marriage counseling session together, I was doing all the talking and Dan would agree to everything I was saying.   Then

I asked Dan to go to counseling by himself because I wanted him to talk to the counselor alone so he could feel comfortable telling the counselor how he was feeling without me judging him.

It was now January, 2008, and because of Dan's work schedule, it made it difficult for Dan to go to counseling sessions alone, so we would go to group sessions together whenever Dan was available. I continued to go to counseling by myself. The counseling helped and soon Dan and I were making progress in getting our marriage back on track. We were sleeping together again and our intimacy was gradually starting to improve. Dan was making an effort to come home at a decent time so we could have dinner together and was working hard on trying to communicate with me.

Things started to improve and by April 2008, I decided to dismiss the divorce proceedings. I can't say that our marriage was back to normal, but it did improve and we were both working hard on making it work. We continued to go to marriage counseling. I believe we went to marriage counseling for about a year or so.

A few months after we stopped going to marriage counseling, Dan began coming home late again and not calling me and we began arguing again.

Soon I was starting to get depressed because I felt we worked so hard in getting our marriage back on track and then Dan starts going back to his old habits of coming home late and not calling me and not communicating with me and that's when I began to stop communicating with Dan and began gambling.

Gambling–my form of self-medication

"Self-medication is a human behavior in which an individual uses a substance or any external influence to self-administer treatment for often unmanaged, undiagnosed physical or psychological ailments."

In layman's terms, it's a way of coping with stresses or conditions that don't seem to be controllable.
Most people think of alcohol or drugs as the coping mechanisms but there are many others including becoming a workaholic, or addictions to sex, exercise, and gambling.

Because I was not getting what I wanted at home, and I was so unhappy, I began going to the Casinos to gamble at least six times a month as a form of compensation for my frustration and a way of coping with the situation.

It got to the point where I would get into an argument with my husband just so that I could leave the house to gamble.

I would be gone all day and sometimes come home late at night.

I would go to Agua Caliente Casino in Palm Desert, Morongo Casino in Cabazon and San Manuel Casino in Highland.

I would spend approximately $300.00 each time I went, and that was only because I could only withdraw $300.00 a night from the ATM machine.

Sometimes I would stay late at the casino so that I could withdraw money after midnight.

I was gambling at least $1,200 a month and Dan had no idea where I was or what I was doing. When I would come home, he would ask where I was all day.

I would reply; it's none of your business, you don't call me when you are going to be late from work, you don't have sex with me anymore, so why should I stay home with someone who does not pay attention to me?

Dan then started to accuse me of having sex with other men and wanted to know where I was.

I would tell him that I wished I had men that would give me what he couldn't give me anymore and that I wished I was that lucky.

All I could think of was, when is the weekend going to get here so that I could go to the Casino and get my adrenalin rush?

I was so depressed that going to the Casino was exciting for me each time I went. I was happy for hours just playing, winning, losing and winning again. This went on for about 6 months.

One time I won $2,100.00 and I was so excited that I didn't know where I had parked my car.

I had to be escorted to the parking lot in a golf cart so I could find my car.

Then one day, I finally had enough of this crazy way of living, and I said to myself, I can't live like this anymore, I have to make a change in my life and in our relationship so I took my friends Rachel's, Bill's and Mike Connolly's advice and scheduled an appointment for Dan to see our primary physician.

Chapter 11

The Reunion

In 1966, when I was five years old, I met my best friend, Rachel Rodriguez. She was Hispanic but looked Caucasian with her fair skin, dark brown eyes and light golden brown hair.

We lived across the street from each other but never really got to know one another until we entered Kindergarten.

I was a skinny Hispanic kid, with long dark brown hair hazel eyes, who barely spoke English. We hit it off right away and she helped my sister and I learn to speak English.

Soon after we would go to each other's house and hang out. We also played outside with a dozen other kids.

We lived on Amethyst Street, a very steep hill in the suburbs of Los Angeles, California, called El Sereno. We knew everyone in the neighborhood, and I mean everyone. Not like today, where you barely know your neighbors or the children on your block.

We would always hang out and played games late at night with the other kids on our block until our parents called us to come inside.

We played a game called "kick the can." For some reason I would always be the one who would get stuck with the can and would have to go looking for the other kids.

It was like hide and seek but every time someone would come out from hiding, they would kick the can and I would have to start all over again looking for my friends.

One time I just gave up, didn't say anything to the kids, and went inside my house. The funny thing is, my friends thought I was still looking for them, but Rachel, who knew me so well, was the only one who figured out that I had gone inside.

Rachel and I did a lot of things together like learning how to ride bikes. One time I went down the steep hill we lived on, crashed and chipped my front tooth. I did not realize I had chipped my front tooth until Rachel started laughing and said "you look like a clown, I told you not to go down that hill."

After the bicycle incident, I was determined to learn how to ride skates down the hill like Rachel and her sister Rita did.

Rachel taught me how to skate in the parking lot of our elementary school and before I knew it, I was skating down the hill with Rachel and her sister.

Our parents would yell at us and say, "Do not skate in the street; you're going to get hurt or get hit by a car," but we didn't listen.

One day when we were skating down the street, a car drove up very fast. Everyone heard the skid sound of the car and ran out of the house to see what happened. The car stopped just in time and missed hitting us.

After that incident, we were not allowed to skate on the street again. I have to say, we were really good. We could have been on Roller Derby, but we were too young.

Rachel was always there for me, even when I was drowning at Pudding Stone Lake in San Dimas. Her parents would take all five of us kids in their 1972 red Volkswagen to Pudding Stone Lake each summer. Rachel's older brothers and their wives would go too.

One summer, I thought I could swim to a floating dock about 20 yards from shore.

Rachel and I were swimming together to see who could get there first. Suddenly, I got tired and realized I didn't know how to float or tread water and began to go under water.

Rachel tried to help but because she was not a great swimmer she couldn't help me. Rachel yelled to her brother Rudy, who was swimming nearby that I was drowning.

While I was drowning, all I could think of were my nieces and family and how I wasn't going to see them anymore if I drowned. Then, I remembered seeing a commercial on TV where the girl dove into the water and moved her hands sideways up and down.

I started to do that but it seemed as if I was doing that forever when all of a sudden I was up to the water's surface.

Rachel's brother Rudy and his wife Irene were there when I came up and attempted to push me to shore. I was in such a panic that I was drowning them too. They finally got me to shore and were relieved that I had not drowned.

All I could think of to say was "don't tell my mom and dad about what happened 'cause they will not let me hang out with you guys again." And then I said, "I'm hungry."

I was no longer scared.

The following summer I learned how to swim and the rest, as you say, is history.

Rachel's parents had three minor children, including Rachel. My sister Margaret and I were like their adopted children and they'd take us everywhere they took their children. We would go to Disneyland once a year, Knott's Berry Farm, the beach, the zoo, to Griffith Park, and other places.

My parents couldn't afford to take us anywhere because they had 8 children to support and barely had enough money to feed and clothe us, let alone take us anywhere, so we were happy to be a part of the Rodriguez family.

Rachel's parents loved us as if we were their own children. They were so good to us and I will never forget them.

The teenage years were fun too. One day, we decided to ditch school and decided to take the bus to downtown Los Angeles. It was my first time ditching and I was nervous about getting caught. Rachel had done it before with my sister Margaret and some other kids and she assured me that we would not get caught that she and the others did it all the time.

Downtown was approximately 4 miles from our high school. During the 4 mile bus ride, I just kept telling Rachel that I did not have a good feeling about this trip. Rachel kept saying "stop it you are going to jinx us."

We finally made it to downtown and as soon as we stepped off the bus, a Truant Officer approached us and asked us what school did we attend? I immediately said Lincoln High School.

The Officer then said, "please come with me." He placed us in the back seat of the car. Rachel then says "stupid, you should have said we went to Catholic School" and I replied, "you're stupid, you didn't tell me to say that."

During the ride to the Truant Office, all I was thinking was that I hoped my father would not find out or else I would be hit with the belt. Rachel was scared too, because if her father found out, she too would get hit with the belt. (In those days we didn't know about the Department of Public Children's Services).

We were taken to see a Truant Judge and our parents were called to come and pick us up.

Because both our mothers did not drive, Rachel's mother called her father at work to drive them to pick us up.

My mother didn't speak English and Rachel's parents spoke Spanish so they explained to my mother what happened and said we were okay, that all they had to do was pick us up from the detention office.

We stood before the truancy judge and received an ear full about how important school was and that skipping school would only get us in trouble and that she didn't want to see us again, otherwise, we would be put in Juvenile Detention Center.

We were both relieved that we didn't get sent to Juvenile Detention Center. We were released to our parents. My mother didn't tell my father so I wouldn't get with the belt. But she assured me that the next time I ditched school, my father would be told.

Unfortunately, Rachel got hit with the belt, because her mother had to call Rachel's father to take my mother and her to pick us up. Rachel wasn't mad at me because she got hit and I didn't. Lesson learned. I never ditched again, at least not on the bus.

While in high school, we learned to drive and took a driver's education class together. We had so much fun learning how to drive and seeing each other make the same mistakes. We would go out on the street and actually drive.

Our instructor would take us up these steep hills where we would take turns driving. I had the biggest crush on our driving instructor. Back in those days there weren't any rules about dating your teacher, at least if there were rules, we didn't know about it.

My instructor was 26 and I was 17. I trusted Rachel and we told each other everything. One day I told Rachel that I was going out with our driving instructor and that he was teaching me how to drive after school.

Rachel said "sure he's teaching you how to drive. Just be careful." She never told anyone about my crush for our instructor or that he was teaching me how to drive after school.

Then something happened; we changed, met boys, and I fell in love.

I spent all my time with new my boyfriend, Richard. He was extremely good looking, 5'8", 130 lbs, hazel eyes, and light brown hair. He was 20 years old. He was my first true boyfriend who owned a car.

I was madly in love with him and was spending all my time with him. I stopped going out with and calling my friends. When Rachel would call I would tell her "I can't hang out I'm going out with my boyfriend."

Before we knew it, we had stopped spending time together, stop going out, and had just stopped talking.

We met in kindergarten and stayed best friends up until high school.

I recall that we had an argument. I don't remember what the argument was about but it was probably something stupid and all I knew was that we parted enemies and we never spoke again.

Although Rachel and I never spoke to one another, we still kept in touch with each other's families. We would see them at family functions or when we visited our parents on Amethyst Street.

I always knew how Rachel was doing because I kept in touch with Rachel's sister-in-law, Rosalie (Rose), who was my best friend and was eight years older than I.

She would tell me everything that was going on with Rachel. I missed Rachel but I was always afraid to call her. I didn't think she would talk to me if I called her because she was so full of herself she would never admit she did anything wrong.

In my late 30s, I found out that Rachel was getting married. Rachel's sister-in-law Rose had invited me to the wedding.

I asked "Is it ok with Rachel?" She said "Yes!" but I didn't believe her so I didn't go.

Rachel was now married and had two boys. I was happy for her, and I missed her. I was too scared to call and didn't know the best way to get in contact with her.

I kept thinking that Rachel hated me and would just hang up if I called, or slam the door in my face if I knocked on her door.

I just didn't know how to approach the problem. But when I stopped and thought about our childhood and all the good times we spent together, I missed her even more. I also wondered if Rachel ever thought about me or if she just forgot about me. For some reason, I would always remember Rachel's birthday and thought of her every year on her birthday, but was still too afraid to call.

In February of 2007, while I was driving home from work, my phone rang and it was Rachel's sister-in-law Rose. She told me that Rachel's dad was in the hospital, and that he had cancer, and wasn't doing well.

I remembered that this was a man who made my childhood so much fun and whom I loved very much. I asked "do you think Rachel would mind if I went to see him?" She said "No! Rachel has changed, she is so nice, I know she won't mind."

I called my sister Margaret to tell her what was going on with Rachel's dad and she said "Let's go." I felt better that my sister was going with me.

I didn't know what to expect even though I heard how nice Rachel was. I never really believed she would talk to me. When we stopped talking we were eighteen years old, we were now in our forties.

A lot of time had passed, I was more mature, but I was still nervous and asked my sister "what if Rachel gets mad or ignores me what do I do?" My sister just said "relax; it will be ok. It's been a long time, I'm sure she's not still holding a grudge."

But all I could think of was what Rachel's reaction would be when she saw me. Would she approach me and say "what are you doing here and what do you want? You don't belong here" and ask me to leave?

On the drive down to the hospital I was quiet and my sister Margaret kept asking me "what's wrong?" I would say nothing. I kept thinking of Rachel's dad and what a wonderful man he was but at the same time I was thinking "is this a good idea?"

Margaret and I loved Rachel's dad because he was so good to us and I thought it was worth the risk. I said "if it turns out bad I'll just walk out."

We finally got to the hospital, took the elevator up to the second floor, and when the door opened we heard people talking. As we walked toward the waiting room I told my sister "it's really crowded."

I thought there were a lot of people here to visit other patients as well, but it turns out all of them were family members of the Rodriguezes, here for Rachel's dad. Some of them recognized us and said hello, but for some reason I didn't see Rachel. I thought she might not be there and then her mother said that she was in the room with her dad.

Margaret and I spoke to Rachel's mom and expressed how sad we were to hear Jorge was not doing well and that we wanted to be here for her and the family. She said she was glad that we came and said we could go see Jorge.

I was still nervous when Margaret and I walked in the room. At first Rachel didn't see me because she had her head down. Rachel had not changed; she still looked the same as she did in high school. When Rachel looked up, she saw me and I saw her. Rachel got up walked towards me, put her arms around me and hugged me. All my fears were gone.

She said "thank you for coming, how did you find out?"

I said that Rose had told me and that she'd said it was okay for us to come down. Rachel then said "of course, thanks for coming."

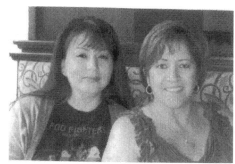

Rachel & Erni

Jorge was sleeping and was unaware that we were there, but we didn't care, we just wanted to be there for Rachel and her family and to see Jorge and tell him that everything would be okay and to hang on.

74

We stayed in the room for a short time and then we waited for Rachel to come out so we could talk. Rachel and I walked to another part of the waiting room so we could have some privacy where she told me all the sad details and that she didn't think her dad was going to make it.

I looked in her eyes and I could see how sad and scared she was. But in her voice I also heard how happy she was to see me. I realized I had to be there for my best friend to get her through the tough times that lay ahead. I just wanted to be there for her, whether it was to hold her hand, listen to her, or whatever she needed. It was going to be hard, but I wanted to be there for her now. We talked every day after that and she would tell me how her dad was doing.

Our reunion didn't feel like a reunion, we both felt like we were never apart. We picked up exactly where we left off 27 years ago, like it was yesterday. We were so happy we were best friends again!

Rachel was at the hospital every day and wanted to be there for her dad when he passed because she didn't think that he should die without one of his family members near.

There were about thirty members in her immediate family and Rachel and her sister Rosic wcrc the only ones there all the time. Rachel could not understand why no one gave a crap. Rachel knew her dad was not doing well and would soon pass away, and she wanted to spend as much time with him as she could.

She didn't care if he didn't know she was there; she just wanted to be by his side in the event he passed away. She didn't want him to be alone when that time came.

Then, on March 2, 2007, Rachel called me and said her dad had passed away, that she was by his side and that he didn't die alone. That was Rachel's biggest fear, for her dad to die alone. Rachel was grateful that she was there with him.

I knew Rachel would take the loss of her dad very badly so I stopped and picked up some pizza, drove down to her home in El Sereno and we talked about what a wonderful dad she had, about our childhood, and how lucky we were to have such a wonderful loving father.

We asked each other why we stopped talking, but neither one of us could remember. We both cried and held each other and I was glad to be there to wipe her tears. I would call and ask if she needed anything but all she would say is No, I have my best friend back, and I'm going to be fine.

At the funeral I sat up front with the immediate family. Rachel read a eulogy that included me in it. It was so beautiful.

Rachel and I had twenty-seven years of catching up to do, and we were on our way. The first question she asked was "why didn't you go to my wedding?"

I started to laugh and told her "I thought you didn't want me there." Rachel replied "of course I wanted you there; when Rose [her sister-in-law] asked if she could invite you I said yes." Rachel told me how much she missed me and how happy she was to see me. I was glad I was there for my best friend during the most difficult time of her life and soon she would be there for me.

Rachel and would try to see each other every chance we could. We were trying to make up for lost time. There is nothing we don't tell each other. Rachel and her husband Craig would go out with Dan and me and we would have a great time. Dan could carry on a conversation and enjoyed talking to Rachel's husband about music and computers, while Rachel and I would play catch up. We didn't always hang out with the boys because they didn't have time, both had jobs with long hours, but when we did get together Dan and Craig had a lot to talk about and we had a great time.

Because we could talk about everything and anything, I called Rachel up to get her opinion on something. I asked "how many times a week do you and Craig have sex?" She was honest and said twice maybe three times a week but lately she'd been tired and wanted to sleep.

"Why?" She asked.

"Because, Dan and I would have sex like four to three time a week, now it's down to once a week and when I tell him "let's have sex" he says "no, I have to get up early for work" or "I'm too tired." He is always making up excuses.

Rachel said well maybe he is tired. I said "all the time?" "We rarely have sex anymore. I like sex, I need sex and I'm going to go crazy if I don't get it." Rachel laughed and said I was crazy.

I asked Rachel "what do you think it could be? Could he be seeing someone else?" Rachel said "No! Dan loves you and I can see it when I'm around you guys." Then she asked me, "Have you asked Dan about it?" "I did," I responded. "He just says he's tired."

Then things started to change. I was getting frustrated with Dan and the no sex thing. I would call Rachel at least once or twice a week crying about how miserable I was and Rachel would always be there for me.

I told her what was going on with Dan and I and that we were not having sex. I told her I thought he was having sex with someone else. But again Rachel was sure he wasn't. Rachel kept telling me to go talk to him but when I did, Dan would say nothing. Dan would look at me as if he didn't understand what I was saying.

It was August 2007, the beginning of Dan's aphasia. One day, I asked Dan to put away some red powdered paint that he had left outside in the back driveway near the garage because I was afraid the dogs would get into it. Dan replied, "Okay."

The next morning, I let the dogs out at 4:30 a.m. to go potty and they didn't come back. I thought that's strange, oh well, they're probably just playing.

When they came back in the dogs were red. I thought they were bleeding but when I got close enough, I saw that it was the red powered paint that Dan left outside. I was mad. Why didn't Dan put it away like I asked him to? I yelled at Dan, "I thought you said you put the powder away." Dan just stared at me with no answer, no expression.

I told him he'd have to go to work late and clean the dogs and the house because they got the red powder everywhere. He said okay and next thing I knew, he was out the door.

I was frustrated and upset and called our dog walker, Donna. I was crying over the phone she said "what's wrong?" I told her what happened and she said "don't worry, go to work, I will pick them up and get them all clean by the time you get home from work."

When I got home, the dogs were somewhat clean, but they still had some of the red powder on their fur. I was so grateful that Donna came to my rescue that I gave her $60.00. Later I called Rachel, told her what had happened, and how frustrated I was with Dan.

She said "Don't be upset. Where can we meet to talk?" "I will meet you wherever you want." I said "okay, I'll meet you at Twohey's in Alhambra."

I told Rachel "I don't know what's going on. He docsn't do what I ask him to do and just ignores me." Rachel said maybe you should take him to see a doctor because this doesn't sound right and just doesn't make sense. This is not the Dan I met, something's wrong." I kept telling her "no he's ok. Maybe he's just tired of me and found someone else."

I've known women whose husbands did the same thing Dan was doing to me; having less sex, ignoring them, and then leaving them for another woman. That's all I could think about, which made me upset and frustrated me even more.

Every time Dan and I argued, which was often, I was doing all the yelling while Dan just stared at me. Once again, Rachel was there for me.

I finally told her I wanted to file for a divorce again but Rachel said "wait before you do it." "Think about it Erni, since I first met Dan I could see how in love he is with you. I can't believe he's fooling around on you and I don't think he's ignoring you on purpose. Go take him to see a doctor, have him checked out, and then if the doctor says everything is ok, then you can file."

Rachel and my niece Nicki were positive that something was wrong with Dan and they believed that Dan was not doing all those things on purpose.
Rachel was adamant that there was something wrong with Dan. I finally took her advice and in October of 2010 scheduled an appointment for Dan to get a physical.

To my surprise Rachel, Nicki, Mike and Bill were right, Dan did have a problem. It was called Primary Progressive Aphasia, and so my story begins.

Chapter 12

How My Relationship With My Family and Friends Helped

Having a support group and a loving family and friends helped me through my depression and frustration.

I don't believe I could have made it without the support from my wonderful and dear friend Marichelle. She was always there for me. I would call her almost every day and night and cry to her about how miserable I was in my marriage to Dan.

I would tell her how he didn't have sex with me anymore, how he didn't pay attention to me anymore and how I was doing everything myself around the house because every time I would ask Dan to do something he wouldn't do it.

It was better to do it myself then to try and get him to do it. Just asking him to feed the dogs and change their water was a task.

I would leave for the weekend and when I would come home the dogs would not have water in their bowls. Taking out the trash was a big deal, too. If I didn't do it, the trash wouldn't get picked up.

Every weekend was one thing or another. I would make plans for us to do something and Dan would tell me at the last minute he had a job to do and wouldn't be able to go with me to a family function or out to dinner.

This would happen on a regular basis, which made me believe he was having an affair. Marichelle would say to me that he was not having an affair and that Dan loved me.

She was there for me too when I filed for divorce in 2007. She knew I didn't want the divorce, and said things will get better, just give it some time. She said Dan was a great guy, who loved me very much, but that we had to work on communicating with one another. I told her it's not me, it's him, he does not communicate with me. She knew our history and knew we both loved each other.

Dan wouldn't respond every time I would bring to his attention to the fact that our relationship was breaking down and he needed to get his shit together or else there wouldn't be "us" anymore.

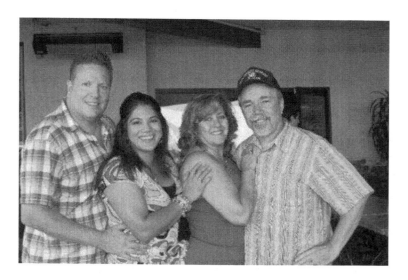

Jack, Marichelle, Erni and Dan

Dan's response would be "okay, let's do it. Let's fix it."
And again it would be the same argument over and
over again. If it wasn't for Marichelle, Nicki, Corina,
Margaret, Rachel and my neighbor Wendy, I may have
had a nervous breakdown or something. It's because of
them that I kept strong and didn't give up.

My niece Nicki would often tell me that Dan was not
ignoring me on purpose and that he loved me. Every
time I would get upset about something Dan did or
didn't do, Nicki would reassure me that he was not
doing those things on purpose and that he loved me.
My friend Corina was very supportive as well, she too
would always be there for me.

She knew how upset I would get every time Dan would
ignore my friends or be rude to her son Kennie. She

would often say I was over reacting and making the situation a lot bigger than it really was, not to let it get to me.

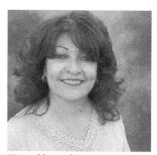

Erni's sister Margaret

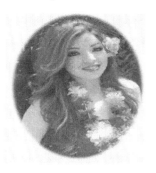

Niece Nicki

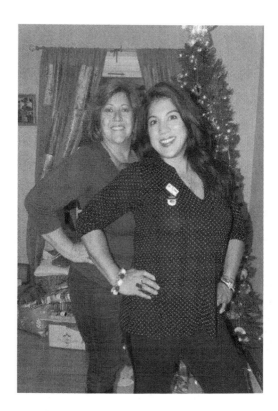

Erni & Marichelle – Xmas 2014

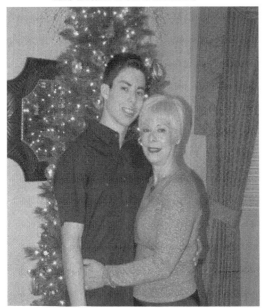

Kennie & Corina

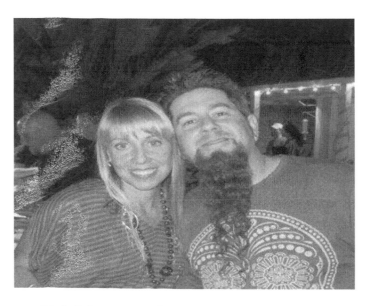

Neighbor Wendy and husband Chris

Ernestina Connolly

Chapter 13

Dan's Family and My Family's Reaction When I Told Them About Dan's Condition

Dan's older brother Mike was working overseas, and the only way to contact him was by email. So I addressed the email to Mike and his wife Debbie.

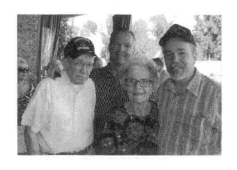

Dan's parents Bill & Rosanna & brother Mike

I explained that the reason Dan and I were not getting along and arguing all the time was because Dan didn't understand what I was saying. This caused him to do all the strange things that he was doing and that I had to learn how to talk to him much slower so he could understand what I was saying.

I gave them the website of the medical condition called Primary Progressive Aphasia so that Mike could look it up and understand what Dan's condition was all about so when he returned from overseas, we could sit down and discuss how best to handle this situation. I also asked him to get his wife Debbie's opinion as to how we could best help Dan.

Debbie's email response was —"I'm sorry to hear about the diagnoses. But at least you now know what you (we) are dealing with. Talk to you soon. Btw, I just tried to call but no one answered."

That was the extent of her email. I was surprised that her email was short and that she didn't try calling me again.

It bothered me for some time and then I realized that I can't expect everyone to feel or respond the way I would so I didn't give it another thought.

When Mike returned from his overseas assignment, he contacted me and asked if I was going to take Dan to get a second opinion. I told him no, that Dan's doctor was a world renowned neurologist and that she had conducted other tests to rule out Alzheimer's, dementia, stroke or a tumor.

Mike expressed to me that he felt Dan was putting in too many hours on the computer both at work and outside of work and said Dan should take it easy. He also felt Dan was under a lot of stress which was probably the cause of his condition, or at least was the beginning of Dan's condition.

He wanted Dan to take time off work or find another job because he knew how hard Dan had been working and the stress that Dan was under. But because Dan was so passionate about his work, there was no way that Dan would take time off, let alone find another job that was less challenging.

I thanked Mike for his opinion and said he was probably right, that Dan was working too many hours and was under a lot of stress.

I don't believe Mike understood how severe Dan's condition was until a year or two later when he finally realized how difficult it was for his brother to communicate and understand what we were saying to him.

Mike loves his brother and would do anything he could for him. Mike also felt that speech therapy would be helpful for Dan. I told Mike that Dan had been seeing a speech therapist twice a month for about a year, which seemed to help.

After the incident that occurred in January of 2014, we couldn't afford for Dan to continue his speech therapy. I had to hire someone to stay with Dan a couple of hours a day and take Dan to get something to eat at lunch time, because Dan wouldn't always eat the food I left for him.

With all due respect to Dan's father, Bill, he didn't say much when he was told about Dan's condition. When I finally asked him about his reaction to Dan's condition, Bill indicated that he was worried about us financially and wondered if we would be able to keep our home should Dan's condition prevent him from working.

He knew how smart Dan was and was confident that Dan would be okay because he had me to take care of everything. Not that everything I did was right, but he knew I would do what was best for Dan and our future.

As for Dan's mother, Rosanna, she was very understanding and was sad that her son was going through this difficult time in his life. At the same time she knew that I loved her son and that I would do whatever it took to help Dan get through this.

Rosanna felt confident that I would know what to do when Dan's condition got worse. She knew Dan was getting the right care he needed and that I would take care of him no matter what.

Dan's daughter Maureen did not quite understand what was wrong with her dad, she believed it was the early stage of dementia and that he would be okay and that speech therapy would make him better. I tried to explain to her that it wasn't dementia but she was in denial. Maureen lived in Arizona and didn't see her dad much except maybe once or twice a year, so she didn't get to see or talk to her dad on a regular basis to recognize how severe his medical condition was.

My entire family was very supportive of what I was going through with Dan and they couldn't imagine how I was dealing with this devastating news. They too loved Dan and were saddened that Dan was going through this.

When my 7 year old nephew, Ryan, found out about his Uncle Dan's medical condition, his mother explained to him that the dictionary in his uncle's brain is not working properly. Uncle Dan has trouble understanding what you are talking to him about so make sure to be nice to Uncle Dan if he doesn't respond.

It's amazing what children remember at a young age. Just a few weeks ago, Dan and I went to see my nephew Ryan, who is now 9 years old, play soccer. Dan never goes anywhere without his camera and proceeded to take pictures of Ryan.

Dan ran across the field to take more pictures of Ryan and when the game was over, Dan had taken lots of photos and showed them to us.

A few days later, my niece called me to say that Ryan told her that his coach was yelling at uncle Dan to get off the field but that uncle Dan didn't understand the coach. Ryan said that he yelled at his coach and said "that's my uncle Dan, his dictionary in his brain does not work and he does not know what you are saying."

The coach said okay sorry, it's okay. That really touched my heart to know that even a young child understands what's happening to Dan and has compassion for him.

Then you have those individuals who don't understand Dan's medical condition, and don't know how to communicate with him and can't help you.

Dan had always taken care of me and I knew that I had to take care of him now. I told my family that I didn't know how I was going to do it, but that I was going to do whatever it took to help Dan with this condition.

I told them that my entire mission in life was to make sure Dan was taken care of and that he is happy and stress free so that he could continue to live the best quality of life that he could.

My family knew what a positive and strong individual I was and that I have always taken charge of whatever situation came my way. They knew I would be okay and that Dan was in good hands.
My sister Margaret was very supportive and was always there to listen to me whenever I got frustrated. She knew how tired I was and all that I was going through. I often stopped by her house on the way home from work to pick up dinner she made for Dan and me.

My mother was sad to hear about Dan's medical condition. She has always liked Dan. Even though Dan didn't speak Spanish, and she didn't speak, English, they both got along.

She was concerned for my health because of my diabetes and felt that the stress of Dan's medical condition might make my condition worse. I assured her that would not be the case, because I was here to stay and to care of my Sweetiepie. She too was glad that I was a strong individual who could handle anything that came my way.

When my brother Rene died at the age of 43 of a heart attack, I was the one who made all the arrangements for his funeral (with the help of my niece). My brother and I were not particularly close, partially because he was either in jail or living on the streets because of his drug use, but I would help him whenever I could. I would buy him clothes, help with his rent, write to him when he was in jail, and send him money so that he could buy cigarettes or whatever he needed that he could purchase at the jail facility.

It wasn't until after his death that I found out that we were so much alike. We both had hazel eyes, loved animals, made friends easily, talked to strangers, liked the same kind of foods, and ate our food exactly the same way by placing everything on a plate and mixing it all together. We liked the same song by Al Green and were always smiling and joking around.

Rene knew my favorite actor was Al Pacino. Before Rene's death he bought me some flowers and gave me a book on Al Pacino. That was his way of thanking me for all that I did for him. He had just gotten out of jail 3 months prior to his untimely death, he had a job and was the happiest anyone had ever seen him.

His death didn't hit me until 3 months later when I was driving to work one day and I was thinking about him and the song by Al Green that we both liked suddenly came on the radio. My tears fell like rain. It was then that I realized that I would never see or talk to him again.

Chapter 14

The Doctor's Appointment

I contacted Dan's primary physician and was able to schedule an appointment for Dan to get a physical on October 9, 2010.

It is now October 9, 2010. Dan and I met with his doctor. I informed the doctor that I felt like I was being a nagging wife because my husband would not pay attention to me and when I'd ask him to do something he says OK, but when I would come home, it would not be done plus, we were not having sex anymore like we used to and that we were arguing all the time.

The first question to Dan was "Do you know your birthday?" and Dan replied "Birthday?" The doctor said "Yes, when is your birthday?" Dan replied "6/15/53."

Then he asked "do you know where you are at now?" Dan replied "In Pasadena." The doctor replied "Yes Pasadena, but do you know the building you are in?" Dan didn't understand the question.

The doctor asked him again "What type of building is this?"

Dan didn't understand the question. The next statement was "I'm going to name a couple of items and I want you to remember what I said." Dan said "okay."

The items were red, nickel, church, table, and rose. The doctor then made small talk with Dan for about a minute and then asked Dan "do you recall the 5 items

I just told you a minute ago?" Dan replied "okay" so the doctor then asked Dan what the items were. Dan could not remember the items. The doctor then asked "Was one of the items a quarter, nickel or a penny?" Dan replied, "a nickel."

The doctor then asked "was one of the items a couch, table or chair?" Dan replied "a table." The next question the doctor asked "was one of the items a gym, school or church?" Dan said "church."

Dan could not recall the other two items.

The doctor then showed him three pictures; one was a lion, one was a camel, and one was a hippo. He asked Dan if he could name the animals.

Dan looked at each animal but could not recall their names. The doctor then pointed to each of the pictures and asked "do you know where they live?"

Dan immediately said that the camel lived in Egypt, the lion lived in Africa, but could not recall where the hippo lived. The doctor then asked Dan to draw a clock and put the time of 2:00 o'clock on it.

Dan didn't understand the question, the doctor told him again to draw the clock. Dan looked at his watch and said "you want me to do this?" The doctor said "yes, draw a clock with 2:00 o'clock on it."

Dan proceeded to draw the clock with 2:00 o'clock on it.

"Perfect" the doctor said. Then he asked him if he knew what Pasadena was best known for but Dan didn't understand the question and said he didn't know. The doctor said "the Rose Bowl and Rose Parade." Dan replied okay.

The doctor then completed Dan's physical and said he was referring Dan to a neurologist, Richard Spitzner, M.D.

I immediately called Dr. Spitzner's office and was able to get an appointment for Dan to see him in 2 weeks.

I was still not sure what was wrong with Dan.

On October 21, 2010, we met with Dr. Spitzner, a 65 year old man who weighed 250 lbs., was 5"7", had grey hair and a beard.

We waited almost 2 hours before we saw Dr. Spitzner. We almost didn't see him because Dan was getting very anxious and wanted to go home.

As we entered the doctor's office we noticed that it was a small office facing west with a brain sculpture on his desk.

Dr. Spitzner apologized for the long wait and said he likes to be very thorough when he meets with his patients. Dr. Spitzner was pleasant to talk to, honest and very straight forward.

He asked almost the same questions the primary physician asked. He asked Dan whether he knew the name of the top of the coffee cup.

Dan said "cup" and the doctor said; "no, what do you call the top of the cup?" Dan didn't have an answer.

The doctor replied "rim" Dan said "okay."

The doctor then placed a writing pen and a pin on his desk and asked Dan to pick up the pen you write with. Dan didn't understand the question.

He asked him again and Dan picked up the writing pen. He then asked Dan a series of questions, some of which he got right and some he didn't understand.

One question he asked Dan was whether at any time he ever wanted to kill himself? Dan looked and me and then looked at the doctor, so I asked if he wanted me to leave so Dan would feel more comfortable answering the questions. The doctor said "no, you stay here."

He then asked Dan the question again. Dan had this look on his face as to say do I really need to respond. The doctor said "please tell me the truth, it is important." Dan replied, "Yes I have." The doctor then replied, "Do you still want to kill yourself?" Dan said "NO."

I was not surprised to hear that, because I was unhappy about our relationship and wanted to end my life as well at one time or another.

I knew how he felt, but to actually say it out loud and tell someone must not have been easy for him.

The doctor then took Dan to another room and continued with his examination. He made sure all his muscles were moving correctly and had him stretch and touch his toes.

The examination took approximately 2 ½ hours. Finally, the doctor said, "I need a urine specimen an EEG and an MRI," and referred us to an office across the street from his building to get the urine specimen.

We had to come back to his office another day to get the EEG and we were able to schedule an appointment for the MRI on November 10th.

After we left the doctor's office, I thought to myself, there might be something wrong with Dan if they are making him take all these tests.

It is now November 10, 2010. We drive to an office in Pasadena where Dan is to get the MRI. Dan is quiet and doesn't ask any questions, he just wanted to know how long it was going to take because he had to be at work by 10:00 a.m. The test took approximately 40 minutes and we were given a CD of the MRI, which I delivered to Dr. Spitzner's office, just a few blocks away.

We met with Dr. Spitzner about a week later to review the results of the EEG, urine test and MRI. I was not nervous and neither was Dan because I guess I was expecting nothing to be wrong.

Dr. Spitzner said the good news was that the EEG and urine test came out fine but the MRI showed a small dot on the left side of the brain. He was unable to determine what that could be so he referred us to Dr. Helena Chui.

While we were sitting in his office, he called Dr. Chui to schedule an appointment for us to see her. Dr. Spitzner indicated that Dr. Chui was a specialist in the field of Neurology at USC, she gets booked up really quickly so when he called Dr. Chui's office he was told her first appointment would be in February, 2011. I said "okay, please schedule it for us."

Dr. Spitzner said he would forward all of Dan's test results to Dr. Chui before our upcoming appointment with her. He assured us that Dr. Chui was a great doctor and that we would be happy with her, and wished us well.

I don't think Dan knew exactly what was going on, so I didn't say anything to him. There was still tension in our home, I guess it was because we didn't know what to expect and Dan had so much work to do.

Our arguments were minimal now, but we were still sleeping in separate bedrooms.

As we approached Christmas 2010, I had a lot on my mind and wasn't in the Christmas spirit so I told Dan to go to his brother's home without me. Dan's daughter Maureen and her son Gino were visiting from Arizona and I made them go together.

I spent Christmas with my parents in Hesperia. I really enjoy spending time with my parents and sisters. My parents had no clue that Dan and I had been having marital problems or that Dan was having tests done.

It is now February 2011 and we finally arrived at Dr. Chui's office at Keck USC Neurology Department in Los Angeles.

We meet with Dr. Chui's assistant, Dr. Freddi Segal Gedan. She is in her mid-50s, 5'2" with long curly grayish black hair and glasses. She was very sweet and was happy to meet Dan and me. She explained that Dan will be meeting with one of the doctors who will be conducting a variety of studies to determine Dan's verbal, comprehensive, and logical thinking skills, etc. and that it would take approximately 4 to 5 hours.

We arrived at the doctor's office at 1:00 pm and when Dan was finished with all the tests, it was 5:00 p.m. Dan was pretty exhausted and just wanted to go home. I told him that we had to see the doctor and that we would go home soon.

We then met with Dr. Chui, a Chinese woman in her mid-60s, 4'9" 130lbs. She was excited to meet us and we sat down and talked. She asked Dan a series of questions, most of which Dan could not answer. I did mostly all the talking. Then we went over his test results and the MRI.

The doctor told us that she was not happy with the MRI and wanted Dan to have a PET scan. She explained that this test would be more detailed in that it will show the different sections of the brain for better understanding.

I asked if she knew what was wrong with Dan and she replied that they were trying to figure that out, but this PET scan will be able to show us more about what's going on in Dan's brain. Or, there was always the option of getting a sample of spinal fluid from his spinal cord, which involves a large needle and is very painful.

I said no to the painful procedure and opted for the PET scan. She said okay, and that she would contact Dan's insurance carrier to confirm they would pay for this type of test.

About a month later, we got a call from Dr. Chui's office to say that the insurance approved the PET scan so she immediately scheduled an appointment for Dan to get the PET scan.

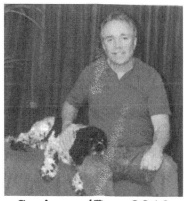

Springer/Dan 2012

It is now the morning of April 7, 2011, Dan and I went to the office in Pasadena, where Dan would be getting the PET scan. We were told that this procedure would only take 40 minutes but whcn we got there we were told that the procedure was actually going to take longer.

I said "okay, we're here so let's do it." Dan still had no clue why he was having so many tests done and I told Dan that this is the last test before we see the doctor again.

Dan and I were called into the office where we met a beautiful nurse named Julie, who explained the procedure to us and advised Dan that he cannot be around children, pregnant women or animals for about 18 hours because he is going to be exposed to radiation.

I said "really? Okay." I then called Dan's work and spoke to his supervisor to say that Dan will not be returning to work today per doctor's orders, but that he will be in tomorrow morning.

He asked if Dan was alright and I replied "yes, he is just having some tests done and the doctor advised him to stay home after the procedure." He said okay and thanked me for letting him know.

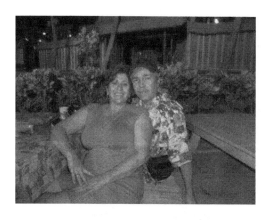

On May 4, 2011, we went to Dr. Chui's office, once again, to get the results of the PET scan.

Erni and Dan in Hawaii 2012

We were escorted to a back room where we were greeted by Freddi who was happy to see us and said that Dr. Chui is running a little late, but she will meet with you.

We talked about how the PET scan went and how Dan was doing since his last visit in February. I told her he is doing okay. When Dr. Chui finally arrived she was happy to see us, as we were to see her.

Dr. Chui asked if we would mind if one of her colleagues joined us during our meeting and I said sure. Dr. Chui asked how the PET scan went and I said it went okay. Then the colleague asked Dan if he could name 4 different animals that had four legs. Dan replied, "You mean Springer, Sportster and ChuChu," I laughed and said those are our three dogs. They all have four legs. Then Dr. Chui said that's right, they all have four legs, that's great Dan.

I had been waiting anxiously for months to find out what was wrong with Dan. We sat down and Dr. Chui turned on the computer in her office.

She began with the phrase, "we have some great news." I said "really, what is it?" Dr. Chui replied, "The results from the PET scan show that Dan DOES NOT have a tumor, Alzheimer's, dementia, nor has he suffered a stroke, which was my concern. However, he does have a condition called Primary Progressive Aphasia, which is what I expected, but wanted to rule out the other conditions."

Dr. Chui turned on the computer and showed us Dan's brain. She began to explain that the left side of Dan's brain was beginning to shrink and that was why he had been having difficulty understanding words.

She said it's like I was talking a different language to Dan. His brain can only remember certain words. She explained that his brain is like a dictionary but the dictionary is not alphabetized so he could only find the words that are floating around in his brain. At some point in time, generally speaking, Dan will not be able to communicate with you.

I began to cry, and asked the doctor, "how can I communicate with him if he can't understand what I am saying?"

The doctor said, "You will find a way." Then she said "what do people from other countries do when they do not speak the same language? Do they just ignore each other, or do they try and communicate by other means? You and Dan will have to get creative in your communications, don't worry, it will be okay."

I'm not sure if Dan really understood what was going on because he was not talking much and I was doing all the talking and asking all the questions. Dan was mostly concerned if he could still work.

The doctor said as long as he felt he was able to do his job and understand what he was doing, he will be okay to work.

I then replied, "Dan's work involves programming and setting up computers for new employees and updating files and data and fixing whatever problems employees are having with their computers. Dan does not have much interaction with co-workers directly, and mostly gets information via email with respect to what needs to be done."

I then asked "what can we do to stop his brain from shrinking" to which Dr. Chui replied "there is currently no cure for Dan's condition, but there is ongoing research."

When I heard "no cure" I thought of cancer and how there is no cure even though there many studies and research being conducted and they still can't figure out how people get cancer or how to stop it from spreading, except with radiation and chemo if they detect it early enough.

This was a totally new disease and only thousands of patients had been diagnosed worldwide with this condition as opposed to millions diagnosed with cancer, MS, Alzheimer's, dementia and AIDS.

I then asked "what can I do to help Dan with this condition." The doctor replied "speech therapy and plenty of exercise and swimming sometimes helps."

I said "Okay, how long can Dan continue to work?"

She said it was up to Dan and how he feels. She explained that this is why his condition is called Primary Progressive Aphasia, because it's progressive, the brain shrinks gradually and that each patient's condition is not the same.

She went on to say "after reviewing Dan's test results, I see that he is a very intelligent man and has an excellent photographic memory. He will be okay, and only Dan will know when he can no longer do his job, but you too need to pay more attention to how he is feeling and if you see any changes in him."

"Because Dan cannot express what he is going through, you will have to be more diligent in recognizing signs that were not there before."
I said "okay, what else can I do" and she replied "you need to see a therapist to help you get through this process; you cannot do it alone." I said "okay, when do I start and how much will it cost?" Dr. Chui said it would not cost anything because it was part of their USC student program. I said "great when can I make my first appointment?"

Chapter 15

Therapy

I began therapy shortly thereafter. I would meet with an intern student from USC for my therapy and he or she would discuss our session with the licensed therapist and go over what we had discussed. Dan too went to therapy, but because of Dan's work hours and schedule, it was difficult for Dan to meet with the therapist on a regular basis.

Talking to the intern really helped me to release the frustration that I was going through and get some answers to the many questions I had about my fears and how to overcome this devastating news and what I could do to better help Dan to get through this.

First, I had to take care of me before I could take care of Dan. I would not be any good to Dan if I wasn't able to deal with what our future was going to be like, because we didn't know.

I had to learn how to accept what Dan was going though and how I could help him get through this to better our lives.

Dan went to a couple of sessions. At one point it was getting difficult for Dan to understand some of the questions and to express how he was feeling or how he was dealing with this condition. Dan stopped going after a few months.

I continued to go 3 times a month. I have to say that it really helped me to talk to someone about what I was going through and the frustrations that I had at times, because it was getting harder to communicate with Dan and I needed someone to talk to let them know how I was feeling so that I did not have a nervous breakdown.

I didn't want my family to know what I was going through because I didn't want them to worry about me. They have enough problems of their own to worry about and because I have always been a strong and positive individual, I knew that I would get through this and be a better wife for Dan and for our marriage.

I did have the support of my family and friends, but sometimes, you cannot tell them everything, as you can a total stranger, who will not judge you for saying what you really feel and what you are going through

I have to say that talking to someone really helped me get through this because there is no wrong answer or right answer, we all learn through experience, trial and error.

We are not perfect and we will make mistakes, but how we deal with them is what matters. So don't be afraid or ashamed to ask for help.

I couldn't have done it alone without the help from the team at USC Neurology.

Ernestina Connolly

Chapter 16

What is Primary Progressive Aphasia (PPA)

As a concerned spouse, I started my own research into Dan's condition.

The following information is what I found and although it may seem a bit overwhelming to read, it doesn't even begin to explain the whole picture regarding the condition, its effects on everybody, including the patient, and the limited research that has been conducted to date.

Primary progressive aphasia (PPA) is a form of cognitive impairment that involves a progressive loss of language function.

Language is a uniquely human faculty that allows us to communicate with each other through the use of words. Our language functions include speaking, understanding what others are saying, repeating things we have heard, naming common objects, reading and writing.

"Aphasia" is a general term used to refer to deficits in language functions. PPA is caused by degeneration in the parts of the brain that are responsible for speech and language.

PPA begins very gradually and initially is experienced as difficulty thinking of common words while speaking or writing. PPA progressively worsens to the point where verbal communication by any means is very difficult.

The ability to understand what others are saying or what is being read also declines. In the early stages, memory, reasoning and visual perception are not affected by the disease and so individuals with PPA are able to function normally in many routine daily living activities despite the aphasia.

However, as the illness progresses, other mental abilities also decline.

Adults of any age can develop PPA, but it is more common in people under the age of 65. People with PPA can have a variety of different language symptoms and no two cases are exactly the same.

Symptoms & Causes

People with PPA can experience many different types of language symptoms.

In many instances, the person with PPA may be the first to note that something is wrong and the complaints may initially be attributed to stress or anxiety.

People with PPA initially experience one or more of the following symptoms:

- Slowed or halting speech
- Decreased use of language
- Word-finding hesitations
- Sentences with abnormal word order in speech or e-mails
- Substitution of words (e.g., "table" instead of "chair")

- Using words that are mispronounced or incomprehensible (e.g., "track" for "truck")
- Talking around a word (e.g., "We went to the place where you can get bread" for the words "grocery store")
- Difficulty understanding or following conversation despite normal hearing
- Sudden lapse in understanding simple words
- Forgetting the names of familiar objects
- Inability to think of names of people, even though the person is recognized
- Problems writing (e.g. difficulty writing checks or notes)
- Problems reading (e.g. difficulty following written directions or reading signs)
- New impairments in spelling
- Problems in arithmetic and calculations (e.g. making change, leaving a tip)

People with PPA tend to have similar clusters of symptoms. Researchers who specialize in PPA currently recognize three subtypes:

1. Agrammatic,
2. Logopenic and
3. Semantic.

PPA-G (Agrammatic/Nonfluent Subtype): A problem with *word-order* and *word-production*

- Speech is effortful and reduced in quantity.
- Sentences become gradually shorter and word-finding hesitations become more frequent,

occasionally giving the impression of stammering or stuttering.

- Pronouns, conjunctions and articles are lost first.
- Word order may be abnormal, especially in writing or e-mails.
- Words may be mispronounced or used in the reverse sense (e.g., "he" for "she" or "yes" for "no").
- Word understanding is preserved but sentence comprehension may suffer if the sentences are long and grammatically complex

PPA-L (Logopenic Subtype): A problem with *word-finding*

In contrast to PPA-G, speech is fluent during causal small talk but breaks into mispronunciations and word-finding pauses when a more difficult or precise word needs to be used.

Some people with PPA-L are very good at going around the word they cannot find.

- They learn to use a less apt or simpler word as well as to insert fillers such as "the thing that you use for it," "you know what I mean," or "whatchamacallit."
- Spelling errors are common.
- The naming of objects becomes impaired.

119

- Understanding long and complex sentences can become challenging but the comprehension of single words is preserved.

PPA-S (Sematic Subtype): A problem with word understanding.

- The principal feature is a loss of word meaning, even of common words.
- When asked to bring on orange, for example, the person may appear puzzled and may ask what an "orange" means.
- Speech has very few nouns and is therefore somewhat empty of meaning.
- However, it sounds perfectly fluent because of the liberal use of fillers.
- The person may seem to have forgotten the names of familiar objects.

Causes

PPA arises when nerve cells in language-related parts of the brain malfunction.

The underlying diseases are called "degenerative" because they cause gradually progressive nerve cell death that cannot be attributed to other causes such as head trauma, infection, stroke or cancer.

There are several types of neurodegeneration that can cause PPA. The two most commonly encountered types are frontotemporal lobar degeneration (FTLD) and Alzheimer's disease (AD).

Both FTLD and AD can lead to many different patterns of clinical impairments, depending on the region of the brain that bears the brunt of the nerve cell loss.

When AD or FTLD attacks the language areas (usually on the left side of the brain), PPA results.

PPA is caused by AD in approximately 30-40% of cases and by FTLD in approximately 60-70% of cases.

In contrast, PPA is a very rare manifestation of AD.

In the vast majority of patients with AD, the most prominent clinical symptom is a memory loss for recent events (amnesia) rather than an impairment of language (aphasia).

PPA is therefore said to be an "atypical" consequence of AD.

The logopenic type of PPA has a particularly high probability of being caused by AD.

Specialized positron emission tomography (PET) scans and examination of the spinal fluid may help to resolve the distinction between the two underlying diseases.

Whether or not PPA is caused by AD or FTLD can be only be determined definitively at autopsy through examination of brain tissue with a microscope.
This can be confusing because for reasons outlined in the previous paragraph, the word "Alzheimer's" can be used in two different ways.

The term Alzheimer's dementia (or Dementia of the Alzheimer-Type) is used to designate a progressive loss of memory leading to a more generalized loss of all cognitive functions.

The term Alzheimer's disease (as opposed to Alzheimer's dementia) is used in a different way to designate a precise pattern of microscopic abnormalities in the brain.

Sometimes these abnormalities become concentrated in language areas (instead of memory areas) of the brain and become the cause of PPA.

So, while PPA patients don't have Alzheimer's dementia, 30-40% may have an atypical form of Alzheimer's disease.

This dual use of the word "Alzheimer's" is confusing, even for the specialist, but is a feature of medical nomenclature that is here to stay.

In the vast majority of individuals, PPA is not genetic. However, in a small number of families, PPA can be caused by hereditary forms of FTLD.

The most common gene implicated in these families is the progranulin gene (GRN).

Other, less common genes implicated in FTLD include the microtubule associated protein tau (MAPT) and a newly discovered gene, chromosome 9 open reading frame 72 (C9ORF72).

Even in families with genetic mutations, one family member may have PPA while others may have behavioral variant frontotemporal degeneration (bvFTD) or movement disorders, including corticobasal degeneration (CBD) or progressive supranuclear palsy (PSP).

In the presence of a genetic mutation, up to 50% of all family members will have FTLD. Therefore, genetic testing is not usually recommended unless several family members have clinical patterns characteristic of PPA, bvFTD, CBD or PSP.

Before proceeding with genetic testing, it's necessary to meet with a genetic counselor to review the implications of the results.

The immediate purpose of genetic testing is to determine whether the person has a mutation that is responsible for the disease. However, the results have profound implications for family members who are healthy, especially those of child-bearing age.

- Do family members want to know the presence of a genetic disease for which there is no treatment?
- Do they realize that a negative result does not rule out the presence of a mutation in another gene not covered by the testing?

Genetic testing for clinical purposes is a serious step that should not be initiated lightly.

Progression

Because PPA is progressive, decline in language ability continues. Additionally, some non-language abilities (memory, attention, judgment or changes in behavior and personality) can be affected.

Disinhibited, inappropriate behaviors (also seen in behavioral variant frontotemporal degeneration) are more common with PPA-S while impairments in problem solving, multi-tasking movement and mobility (of the type seen in CBD and PSP) are more common in PPA-G.

The rate of decline is variable from person to person and unfolds over many years. It is unclear why some people progress more rapidly than others.

Aphasia Definition and how it manifests itself: Currently, there is Limited information based on its rarity.

PPA is caused by degeneration in the parts of the brain that are responsible for speech and language

Why it occurs

PPA arises when nerve cells in language-related parts of the brain malfunction.

The underlying diseases are called "degenerative" because they cause gradually progressive nerve cell death that cannot be attributed to other causes such as head trauma, infection, stroke or cancer. There are several types of neurodegeneration that can cause PPA. The two most commonly encountered types are frontotemporal lobar degeneration (FTLD) and Alzheimer's disease (AD)

Ernestina Connolly

Chapter 17

Could Dan's Condition of PPA Be Caused by "Blue Water" Agent Orange?

It wasn't until recently, September 13, 2014, that I learned about the possibility of Dan being exposed to *"Blue Water" Agent Orange.* Dan served in the U.S. Coast Guard during the Vietnam ("Nam") War.

Dan and I were vacationing in San Diego, California on September 13, 2014, at Coronado Island. We were celebrating our 8th wedding anniversary a month early.

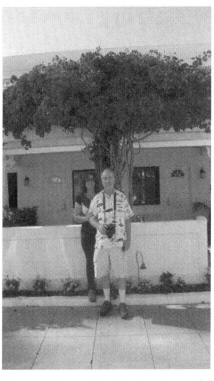

We stayed at the Glorietta Bay Inn, which is one of our favorite hotels on the island.

The Glorietta Bay Inn is a beautiful and famous mansion which was built in 1908 at a cost of $35,000. John Dietrich Spreckles (the Spreckles Sugar Company) designed and built the mansion, which is situated right across the street from the famous Hotel Del Coronado, which was built in 1888. We love to stay there because of its location, history, charm, great price, and excellent hospitality.

Dan and I had booked a 2 hour boat tour the day before to see the north and south sides of the Island.

Coronado Island is approximately 7.9 miles and in the twelve years we had visited Colorado Island, we had never seen the entire island. Since it was going to be a super warm day, I thought it would be nice for Dan and me to enjoy the spectacular view of San Diego Bay.

It was 8:30 a.m. on Saturday morning, and we were waiting for the bus shuttle to take us to the ferry landing which involved a six minute bus ride and about a 20 minute walk from the hotel we were staying.

While we were waiting for the shuttle, we met a couple who were also waiting for the shuttle to take them to the ferry landing.

Since I always talk to strangers, no matter where I go, I introduced myself and Dan and informed the couple that the bus would not be here until 9:00 a.m. and that we had to be at the ferry landing to take the boat across to San Diego by 9:30 sharp. Their names were Marty and Jim.

Marty and Jim were from Ohio and were in Coronado to celebrate the wedding of Marty's daughter. Marty indicated that her daughter would be getting married at the Hotel Del Colorado later that evening.

I congratulated them and said the Hotel Del Coronado was a great place to get married, and that Dan and I had gotten married on the beach in front of the Hotel Del Coronado 8 years ago this coming October.

Marty proceeded to tell me that her daughter was getting married in the small garden part of the hotel and had invited 30 guests to attendance. I told her that the Hotel Coronado was a beautiful place to get married and that I have seen many wedding take place during our trips to the island.

When we got to the ferry landing, Jim decided to get the boat tickets for all four of us to save time, since we barely made it because the bus was late. I thanked Jim and paid him for our tickets when we boarded the boat. We sat next to each other on the way to the other side of the island which took approximately 15 minutes.

During our ride over to San Diego Bay, Jim noticed Dan had a cap on his head that read U.S. Coast Guard Veteran. Jim began to talk to Dan and I indicated to Jim that Dan had a medical condition called Primary Progressive Aphasia and was unable to understand what he was saying.

Then Jim asked whether Dan had been tested for Agent Orange. I told Jim that Dan didn't fight in Vietnam but that he served in the U.S. Coast Guard and was stationed in Wake Island.

Jim then replied, "he didn't have to fight in Vietnam to be exposed to Agent Orange, he just had to be on a ship during 1969 and 1975."

He said for me to look it up on the internet when we got home and to check the va.gov website for more information about *Blue Water Agent Orange.* I thanked him for the information and said our goodbyes.

When we got to our hotel room that evening, I contacted my friend Rachel and told her about what Jim had told me and asked her to look up *Blue Water Agent Orange.*

A few minutes later, Rachel called and said yes, the VA had an article about *Blue Water Agent Orange.* She gave me the website for me to look for myself.

After reading more about Agent Orange, I strongly believe that there is a connection between men and women who served in Nam who were exposed to Agent Orange, sometimes called "Blue Water" Agent Orange or some other type of chemical pesticides which the Government exposed our loved ones to during the Nam War.

I don't believe that it is a coincidence that Dan, and several other servicemen who served in Nam, have the same condition.

In order to get the government to look into this, we need to find more individuals who served in Nam who have PPA. That will be my next mission.

Ernestina Connolly

Chapter 18

Who is Likely To Contract PPA?

This condition affects both men and women between the ages of 40 and 65. It is rare, but some children beginning at the age of 10 can sometimes begin with signs of this condition.

The warning signs

- Non-social behavior; at first you think the person has a hearing problem because you have to repeat yourself a couple of times before they understand what you are saying;
- Then communication starts to breakdown
- Misuse of words when talking
- Repeating the same word over and over again
- Simple tasks are difficult to complete
- Lack of concentration and frustration start to occur
- Their ability to spell words declines

The chronology of the disease

At first, you don't know what's happening to you. You know there is something wrong, but can't put your finger on it. You start to think, is it the stress you are under that is causing you to forget to do things or remember the names of people, places and things?

Then you start to forget the names of cities and states you visited or places you traveled, or the name of a specific band or artist, or the names of the songs you like to listen to.

Before you know it, you can't remember a lot of things and don't know how to explain what's happening to you.

Because of Dan's condition, he is now very limited with names of people, places, and things. He cannot tell you his mother's name or his daughter's name, or the names of our friends and family members, but he does recognize them when he sees them.

He can tell you which freeway to take and can direct you to where he wants to go, or how to get to his parents' home or brother's home or my family members' homes, by just saying left or right and hand movements to go straight.

He can direct you how get home no matter where you are in California.

Watching TV is a challenge for Dan because he is unable to understand what they are saying. Dan only watches Jeopardy® and Wheel of Fortune®. He knows what time they come on in the evening and makes sure we go into the bedroom at 7:00 p.m. to watch the two shows.

Although Dan is unable to understand what they are saying, he enjoys watching the contestants win money and gets disappointed when they lose money, especially when they hit Bankruptcy while spinning the wheel on Wheel of Fortune.

Dan still enjoys listening to music and enjoys watching the PBS station because of the variety of music they offer.

Manifestations of PPA–Where it starts

It begins with a lack of understanding and the accompanying frustration.

For the person with PPA

For the person dealing with PPA they too don't understand what is happening to them so they hide it from their loved ones and employer for fear of losing their job or their loved ones treating them differently.

In Dan's case, he recognized early on that something was not right, but didn't know how to tell me he was having a problem.

He thought maybe he was working too much and it was the stress of his job that was making him forget things that used to come naturally for him.

He'd pretend he was listening to you by saying "okay, that's great," and nodding his head, when in reality, he would only understand half of what you were saying and he had to figure out what you wanted him to do or what needed to be done.

This made it difficult for him to complete the task you or his employer gave him. Dan was good at making believe he understood what you wanted him to do and then when it didn't get done, he couldn't figure out why you were upset.

Dan became depressed as well because we were constantly arguing and I blamed him for our relationship breaking down. Plus, he didn't understand why I was treating him the way that I did and why I resented him.

He would sit in his office at home and stare at the computer for hours. He sometimes wouldn't eat if I didn't have dinner with him, which was often, because he would always come home late from work so I would often eat out or eat alone at home.

In his mind, he was working hard to make the mortgage on our home and to afford us the life style we had adopted; like taking vacation trips twice a year and buying the things we both wanted. He didn't understand why I was always so upset.

Most of Dan's time was spent alone at home, which probably made him more depressed because he did not have anyone to talk to. He was not close to his brother Mike so he couldn't call him to tell him what was going on in our relationship or even ask for advice.

Dan's daughter Maureen lived in Arizona and he didn't want to get her involved in our marriage problems.

Dan was and is a very private person and does not like to discuss our personal life with anyone, let alone talk to his mother or father about our relationship. I'm sure this too was making him more depressed, not having anyone to talk to, because he couldn't even talk to me.

When I think back of how sad and depressed Dan was and how miserable we both were, it breaks my heart to know that I caused so much pain and heartache to the person I love. But then, I tell myself not to let it upset me too much because I didn't know Dan had a medical problem that was causing him to act the way that he did.

Now that I know more about Primary Progressive Aphasia (PPA) and what Dan went through, I want to make our lives as happy and simple as possible. My main concern and goal is for Dan's life to be as normal as possible, to make him happy, and to educate the world about PPA in an effort to find a cure.

For the spouse or partner

As for me, all I was thinking about was that he is not the man I married. It's very frustrating when you are unable to communicate with your spouse.

In the beginning, I remembered thinking he had a hearing problem, but he wouldn't go to the doctor. He would say that he did not have a hearing problem.

Then, it was the lack of intimacy. He would use the excuse that he was too tired when in fact, although that was partially true, the other factor was that he was having trouble getting an erection and didn't know how to tell me.

The most frustrating thing for me was lack of communication and trying to make him understand what I was going through.

An added problem occurs when the other party doesn't understand what you are trying to say and agrees with what you are saying just so that you don't get in an argument.

Many other factors are added to the mix like no longer complimenting you and telling you that you look great or offering a simple thank you for making a wonderful dinner.

I felt like I was not being appreciated for all that I was doing. I was managing the household and at the same time starting a new job and trying to refinance our home.

Then when you find out what the problem is, you have the fear of losing your home and what are you going to do when he is unable to work anymore?

Who will care for him, can you afford to stay home with him, and will you be able to get the help you need when that time comes?

It is a lot to go through, but with the help of family, friends, and a therapist, you will be able to get through it.

The tough part is when you don't have the resources to help you get through this and you are doing this alone.

For the family and friends

It's difficult for family and friends because they don't understand what is happening to your spouse. In the beginning stages, they think he is not sociable and doesn't want to spend time with them.

In some cases, they don't believe there is anything wrong with the person because he looks normal and seems to understand what you are saying.

Only after years of this condition do they start to realize that there is definitely something wrong with him because by this point, he has no clue what you are talking about.

In Dan's case, because we didn't see his family on a daily basis, they didn't see the changes in him, but once they recognized that he had a medical problem, they had a better understanding of what I was going through.

As for my family and friends, they saw Dan on a regular basis so they were able to see the changes in him.

The support of our family and friends is very important on how well Dan does because their understanding of his condition will help Dan to feel comfortable when he is trying talk to them.

If Dan does not feel comfortable talking to you, or if he feels you don't like him, he will not make an effort to talk to you. Being around Dan often, he will feel comfortable around you and you too will feel comfortable around him and will get to know his language.

Just the other day, we were visiting a very good friend of ours, Marichelle. She happened to be taking pictures with a camera Dan told her to buy a couple of years ago. Dan made a comment in his own words and asked whether the 10X camera he told her to buy years prior was still working well for her. She said yes, that it was working perfect and Dan's reply was great, I ordered for you. Marichelle smiled and gave Dan a big hug and said yes, you ordered for me and it was perfect.

What I also want to address is that some family and friends, especially those who are not around your loved one on a regular basis, will not be able to communicate with him or her or may not have the patience to understand what he or she is trying to say.

They may totally ignore him or her or may make comments that will upset you. Don't let what they say or do upset you. Address the issue when it is appropriate and let him or her know how you feel.

Often times when we get upset about how someone treats a loved one with PPA, we want to protect your him or her and may want to verbally attack the person who treated the loved one differently.

Believe me, this will happen and you need to be prepared for when it does. You have enough stress dealing with everyday life, letting an individual get to you is not worth the stress or headache. If they continue to behave in that manner, disassociate yourself with the individual(s) so that you don't have to defend your loved one every time he or she may do or say something that will get you upset. What I say about those types of individuals is that they are ignorant or maybe they lack the compassion to understand you and your loved one and are not worth your time or headache.

Cautions when the symptoms appear

My number one tip is to avoid bad advice from family and friends!

Some family members and friends told me that this was not unusual behavior because their husbands didn't listen to what they would tell them to do either. They said that they too had to constantly remind them to pick up the clothes from the cleaners or not to forget to unlock the gate because the gardener was coming.

They too had to remind them to take out the trash and not to forget that they were going to a family function and not to leave or make any other plans.

Some of my friends and family told me that their sex lives diminished after marriage and I should not expect mine to be any better.

But the difference between them and us is that they have small children or a young teenager at home that causes a built in distraction, so don't believe everything they say.

If something doesn't feel right then go to the doctor and find out what the problem is.

If you happen to have a friend or relative who is negative about your relationship and tries to encourage you to leave your partner so that you can spend more time with them, get rid of the bad apple immediately and get some new friends.

Do NOT make guesses or assumptions based on misdiagnosis or flawed information.

Because this condition is so rare, it sometimes gets misdiagnosed as dementia, Alzheimer's or some form of depression.

Don't take everything someone tells you literally. Do your homework and research your concerns. Talk to your doctor and if he or she does not understand, get another opinion.

Don't give up. Search for more answers if you are not happy with the results you get.

Ernestina Connolly

Chapter 19

The Dog Bite Incident

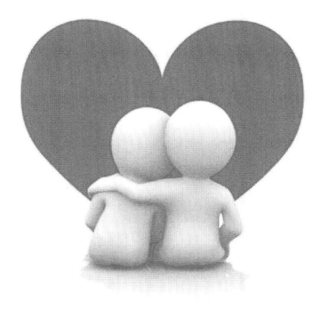

In December of 2013 I dropped our two dogs off at **Petco**® to get a haircut. Dan and I stopped to get something to eat on our way back to pick up the dogs.

Dan placed some leftovers on the floor of the front seat of the car. When he placed our dog Springer in the front seat, Springer immediately got into the small container that Dan left on the floor. Dan went to get the other dog and when he tried to get into the passenger's side of the car, I told him to wait and not to move the dog while he was eating.

I yelled at Dan to stop and not to get the dog when all of a sudden the dog bites his hand. Dan got upset and hit the car door really hard and began to shout "why did the dog do an error for me?"

I told him "I told you not to move the dog but you didn't listen." I finally got the dog in the back seat and attempted to go into the **Petco**® store to get Dan a band aid or something to stop the bleeding. Dan got in the car but didn't understand why the dog bit him. I tried to explain but because of Dan's condition, he had no clue why the dog bit him. When we got home, Springer was so scared from Dan yelling that he went underneath the bed. Later that evening, Dan talked to him like nothing happened.

On May 25, 2014, it is Sunday morning and Dan wanted to take our three dogs for a walk up Azusa Canyon. I said "okay" and proceeded to get the dogs into the car.

I let ChuChu the poodle in first, and then I let Springer in second. I placed Springer (the most aggressive of the three) in the back seat and he immediately started to growl at the poodle. I got into the back seat of the car and tried to calm Springer down. I didn't want the dogs to fight, when all of a sudden Dan approached the car with the third dog (Sportster).

I told Dan not to let the dog in the car because Springer was upset, Dan didn't understand and proceeded to place the dog in the back seat, when all of a sudden, Springer lunged at Sportster and when I went to grab Springer by the collar to pull him away from Sportster, all of a sudden Springer bit my wrist and did not let go.

I finally got my hand free from Springer's mouth and grabbed Sportster out of the car. Dan was just standing there watching me scream.

I told Dan that I was bleeding and to get a towel from inside the house. Dan just stared at me and did nothing. I showed Dan my hand and that it was bleeding because Springer bit me but still got no reaction from Dan.

I finally got the water hose and rinsed the blood from my wrist. Dan replied "let's go to the top." I said no, I have an error and showed him my wrist, but still no reaction from Dan.

I told Dan to take the dogs inside, that we were not going to the top, and that I was going to the doctor to get my error fixed.   Dan said okay, but still had no clue that I was injured.

I got to Urgent Care, which is about 3 minutes from our home, and began to cry, not because it hurt or because of what Springer did, but because Dan had no clue that I was bleeding and he couldn't help me.

I thought "what if I was dying, would he be able to help me?" Probably not and that's what got me upset.   I wasn't even upset that the dog bit me because I knew he didn't do it on purpose, he was just trying to bite Sportster because he didn't want him in the back seat with him.

I came back from Urgent Care and showed Dan my wrist. I tried to tell him that I had an error, but he still did not have any reaction.

I was now worried about what the future would be for Dan and myself if he is unable to recognize danger or I am hurt.

Chapter 20

Doctor's Misdiagnosis of PPA

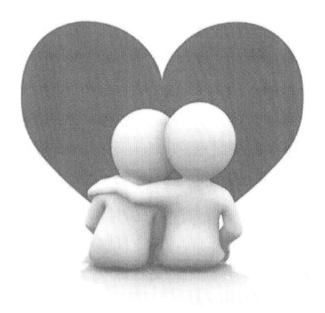

Because the condition of Primary Progressive Aphasia is uncommon, unless you are first seen by a neurologist, it could takes months or years before you get the proper diagnosis.

Many doctors may misdiagnose the symptom as psychological. I say psychological because, often times, people who have this condition are extremely stressed out and have so much going on in their lives that you don't know if it is work related, marital problems, or a mid-life crisis.

Some people get severely depressed because they too don't know what's happening to them.

Many doctors feel that if you are going through some financial crisis, marital problems, or work related issues, that that could be the cause as to why you are reacting or behaving in the manner that you are, so they recommend that you see a therapist.

Another misdiagnosis could be if you are having problems sleeping or sleeping too much and losing or gaining weight and becoming non-sociable.

These could also be a sign that you are depressed and recommendations might include getting psychotherapy and prescribing anti-depressant medication to help you cope with whatever you are going through.

But the medication they prescribe may not always work and sometimes the medication can make you worse, so they try another medication until they get it right. The problem is that by that time, your condition may have worsened and you start to develop other medical conditions such as a stroke or dementia.

The person with PPA may start doing things they have never done before like forgetting to call you when they are going to be home late from work, not remembering your birthday or upcoming events or even the holidays.

People who are overly stressed out don't think about those things. They are so focused on what they are doing that they don't think of anything else but getting the job done, when it may actually be the beginning of the Aphasia progression.

We all tend to forget how to spell a word from time to time but when it happens often, you know there is a problem but don't know how to explain it, what you are going through, and you begin to feel depressed. Often times you don't want to admit to yourself that you are depressed because you don't want to go on some type of prescribed anti-depressant medication.

All these factors come into the equation in determining whether you are actually depressed and going through some mid-life crisis or if you have PPA.

The only way to find out if you have PPA is to have the proper tests done, and unless you have a well-qualified primary physician who can refer you to the right doctor, it could take years to diagnose the condition of PPA.

The first test would be to see a neurologist who will send you to get a MRI, urine test, and EEG. Once you do that, and if it the results come out negative, the doctor may feel you are dealing with depression. You have to remember, the MRI may not show what's going on in your brain because it may be just the beginning so there is nothing there.

Because this condition is progressive, the MRI will eventually show that there is something wrong. Often times, the doctor does not recommend an MRI because you do not have signs of severe headaches; you haven't had a severe blow to the head or severe trauma to the brain so there is no reason to get an MRI.

Having the right doctor who knows what to test for is very important. However, if you are not satisfied with the results, get a second opinion and see another doctor. Also, do your own research on the web.

Being referred to Dr. Helena Chui made all the difference in the world, and although there is currently no cure for PPA, it is a first step in recognizing the condition. Finding more patients with this condition will be the key in getting more research so that we can find a cure.

Chapter 21

The Seminal Event That Led To Understanding the Reality of PPA Costa Rica

After getting the news from the doctor about Dan's condition in May of 2011, I wanted to plan a trip to somewhere we had never been. I asked my best friend, Marichelle, and her husband, Jack, to join us.

They gladly agreed and we immediately made reservations to visit Manuel Antonio in Costa Rica in September 2011. We counted every day before our trip and before we knew it, September 14th was here and we were all packed and ready to go.

Because I was not sure how much Dan understood about his condition, I didn't know how this trip would turn out.

We were in line at the airport checking in and the attendant asked Dan to walk through the X-Ray machine.

Dan looked at me and then the attendant asked whether Dan spoke English. I replied, yes, but he has a disability and did understand your question. I grabbed Dan's hand and moved him towards the X-Ray machine and told him to go through.

When Dan went through it, Dan looked at the attendant and said, "I'm a U.S. Citizen and you don't know what you are talking about." I hurried Dan to the bench to put his shoes on and was praying that he didn't say anymore that could get us put into a room for questioning.

We made it to the terminal and Marichelle and Jack were already there waiting for us. Dan was surprised to see them there. I told Dan they were going with us to Costa Rica, and he replied "really, that's great."

I had indicated to Dan that Marichelle and Jack were going with us, but I guess it didn't register until he saw them at the airport.

The flight was 5 hours long and we had a smooth ride.

When we arrived at San Jose Airport in Costa Rica, we had to take another flight to Manuel Antonio. We were not aware that the flight we were taking from San Jose was a small commuter plane, which holds only 12 passengers.

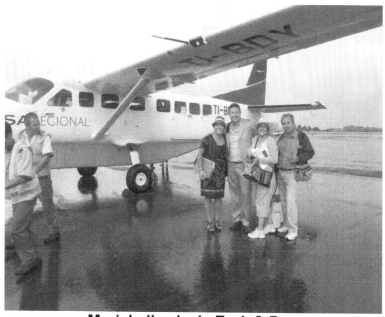

Marichelle, Jack, Erni, & Dan

We were all nervous because the plane was so small and it was raining and overcast. You could not see the sky. The flight to Manuel Antonio was 30 minutes, across the mountains. Jack, Marichelle, and I were nervous about getting on the plane. The pilots were young, probably in their late 20s. Dan was not nervous.

We got into the plane and I sat in the front seat near the window. Dan, Marichelle, and Jack sat behind me.

It was raining and thundering and we all said a prayer that we make it over the mountains. We took off and before we knew it, we were above the clouds and headed towards the mountains.

The pilot assured us that it was safe to fly under these conditions, and that the plane was equipped with sophisticated instruments that show them how far they are from the mountains so that they do not run into them.

I could see the screen on the dashboard with the color "RED" which meant to stay away from the mountains.

I didn't want to see the dashboard anymore and turned to Dan to see how he was doing. He gave me a dirty look and I said "what's wrong?" He didn't answer. When we landed, I asked Dan why was he upset and he said because I didn't sit with him. He was upset for a while until we got to the hotel.

The drive from the small airstrip to our hotel was approximately 45 minutes. The hotel was up on a hill overlooking the ocean below. It was beautiful, just like we saw it on the internet. We were all happy that we made it to the hotel because we were all worried we wouldn't get there. We were shown to our rooms and later met downstairs for cocktails. We had dinner at the hotel because we were too tired to go out. Dan was in a better mood.

The restaurant was quiet and there were only a few other people. We met a woman and her daughter who were having dinner at the hotel that evening because they were leaving for home in Arizona the next morning and didn't want to go out. They told us that they had a great time and that we would enjoy our stay there.

We met a couple of young guys who were also having dinner at the hotel; they were old friends from college and were there for the surfing. They had to get up early the next morning so they could catch the waves.

They told us about a great bar that we had to go before we left Manuel Antonio. They indicated that the bar had a live band and that the drinks were great. We said okay and that we would go there tomorrow. Dan was quiet all through dinner, but loosened up afterwards.

We all put our bathing suits on and headed for the Jacuzzi. It was a long trip and we were exhausted and wanted to relax.

We opened a bottle of champagne and toasted to a great time in Costa Rica. To my surprise, Dan was in the mood for number 3, so I told my friend Marichelle to get lost for a few minutes so that Dan and I could have some fun. Marichelle knew Dan and my history of non-sex in our relationship and gave me a big smile and said enjoy.

The next morning we all got up and had breakfast on the terrace and took a cab ride to the beach. We walked around the small town and then proceeded to hit the beach.

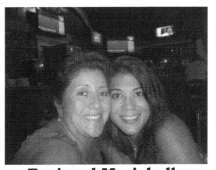

We relaxed and enjoyed our beers on the beach, later Marichelle and I

Erni and Marichelle in Costa Rica

went shopping while the boys stayed at the beach making small talk.

When we got back, we were all hungry and headed to a restaurant where they served the best fish in town. While at the beach we me a woman who was vacationing at Manuel Antonio by herself and we asked her to join us for dinner.

She was delighted that we invited her and we all had a great meal and some fabulous mixed drinks. It was happy hour so we ordered 2 drinks each and before we knew it, we were all laughing and having a great time.

The next couple of days were fun. We went ATC riding to the waterfalls and went on a boat to a snorkeling expedition.

The entire time Dan didn't say much, but I could tell he was enjoying himself and when he did say something it would be "what going on," like he didn't know where we were.

He also would walk in the middle of the street instead of the side of the road. This made me nervous because I was afraid he would get hit by a car, but all he kept saying is that he knew what he was doing.

We only had 2 days left and we decided to go to the rain forest where we could see spider monkeys, sloths, raccoons, and various species of birds and butterflies. At the end of our walk through the rain forest, we ended up on a private beach.

There were signs all over that said **DO NOT FEED THE ANIMALS.**

Of course, Dan didn't listen and when he was taking pictures of the raccoon, he approached the raccoon and bent

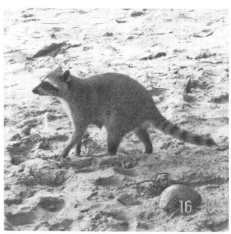

The Costa Rican Raccoon

down to take its picture with a snack bar in his hand.

The next thing you know, Dan comes out from behind the trees and shows my friend Marichelle that his hand is bleeding.

Dan does not react or panic. Marichelle grabs his hand and takes him to the water to wash it down. I was in the water swimming and Marichelle yells at me to come to shore. When I get to shore, I see that Dan has an open wound to his hand. Right away I think "I hope the Raccoon does not have rabies."

We called the park ranger and he called for help. He assured us that the raccoons in the rain forest do not carry rabies, and said Dan needed medical attention to close the open wound and that he should get a tetanus shot.

We finally made it back to the pharmacy, but they were unable to help us. They did not have the tetanus shot available and said we had to go to the emergency clinic.

Lucky for us, the taxi cab driver we used the night before happened to see what was going on and drove Dan and I to the local doctor's office to get stitches on Dan's hand. Dan was so calm about everything and kept saying that he was normal. I said no, we have to get this taken care of.

We finally made it to the doctor's office. It was a small blue home in a residential area that was converted to an office. It was located 30 miles from the beach.

We knocked at the door and there was no answer. The taxi driver called the number that was posted outside the small office and was able to contact the doctor. We waited a few minutes before the doctor arrived.

The doctor spoke only Spanish and asked whether Dan was in a pain. Dan said no. He stitched Dan's hand and referred us to the local emergency hospital which was another 20 minutes away so that Dan could get a tetanus shot. The cost to get Dan stitched up was $100.

We sat in the emergency room for two hours before we were seen. The emergency facility looked like the ones you see in movies. Old and run down, just enough lighting, and short staffed. We finally saw the doctor, who looked at Dan's hand and then called the nurse so that she could inject Dan with the tetanus shot.

The emergency doctor visit cost $180.00 Dan kept on saying he was normal and wanted to go back to the hotel.

It was now 7:00 p.m. and the taxi cab driver came to pick us up. He took us to a restaurant where Marichelle and Jack were waiting for us.

Dan was so calm and did not have a care in the world, he just keep saying "what's going on?" every now and then. We had dinner and then headed for the hotel.

While at the hotel, Marichelle, Jack, and I decided to go to the pool and relax in the Jacuzzi. Dan didn't want to go and stayed behind in the room.

When I came back to the room, Dan showed me his hand. He said it looked bad so he took the stitches off and asked for a Band-Aid.

I said "what are you doing, I just paid $300.00 for someone to stitch you up and you do this?" All he said was that he was normal so I gave him the Band-Aid and we went to sleep.

The next morning Dan was normal, no pain, and he wanted to go home. I told him that we were going home tomorrow and that we were going into town to do some more shopping before we leave. Dan said okay and we all got in a cab and went into town for some more shopping.

Dan kept on opening the Band-Aid to see the cut on his hand. I told him to leave it alone before it gets infected and he kept saying that it was normal.

I didn't want to argue with him so I left him alone and we tried to enjoy our last day in paradise.

Chapter 22

My Worst Fears Came True

On January 16, 2014, at 6:30 a.m., I received a call from my friend Rachel, who told me the hills above our home in Glendora were on fire. I said really, I didn't know, she said "Yes, silly, turn on the news, I believe the fire is right off of Grand Avenue, isn't that where your house is?" I said yes and thanked her for letting me know.

I immediately turned on the news and saw that in fact the fire was burning about a mile from our home. I walked to the front door of our home and could see the flames. I showed Dan the fire and told him that he could not take the dogs up to the canyon (I said you cannot go up on top with the dog). Dan responded "okay."

I wasn't sure if Dan actually understood how dangerously close the fire was to our home. His reaction when I showed him was "the fire was doing east" and I said yes it is.

I was not concerned that the fire would reach our home because it had just started and I thought the fire department would have it out by the time I got home from work.

When I got to work, my co-workers informed me that the fire was getting out of control and that it had burned 20 acres since I left my home just a half hour earlier. I called my neighbor Wendy and told her that if the city called for an evacuation of our neighborhood to get Dan to leave with her and to call me and that I would leave work and meet them. Wendy indicated that she didn't think our neighborhood would be asked to evacuate, but that in the event it did, she would make sure to get Dan and call me.

I watched the news on our office TV and heard the fire was spreading uphill towards Azusa Canyon away from Glendora and by 1:00 p.m. the fire had already burned 120 acres. I was relieved that we didn't have to evacuate our home.

When I got home from work, the fire had consumed over 900 acres and many of the homes above Sierra Madre Blvd. were evacuated, as well as some of the homes in Azusa. I called my girlfriend Corina, who owned a home near Azusa Canyon and asked if they had to be evacuated. She said not yet, but that the fire was getting close to their home and that they were not letting anyone up Azusa Canyon.

The "Coby" fire, as the city called it, burned for about 5 days, when they finally had it contained it had burned 5 homes in the City of Glendora.

A week later, January 24, 2014, was the day I knew would someday come.

I had always prayed that if Dan ever got pulled over by law enforcement, that he would know what to do. I had always told Dan to wear his identification tag on his neck, in the event he would get pulled over and was unable to communicate with the officer, to show them his medical identification tag.

I was at work when I received the phone call from Officer Gibson. It was 12:59 p.m.

Our receptionist, Lenielle, said that an Officer Gibson was on the phone for me. My first reaction was someone was playing a joke on me. At first, I didn't want to take the call and Lenielle said its Officer Gibson and you have to talk to him.

I said okay put him through. The Officer asked if I was Mrs. Connolly and I said yes, Ernestina Connolly. He then said "your husband was in Azusa Canyon with the dog and got in some trouble but he is okay." My heart was pounding but I remained calm.

I immediately thought "did he hit someone on a bicycle while driving up the canyon?"

The officer said that he was taken to Foothill Presbyterian Hospital for observation, but that he was okay. Then the officer said that he might be charged with resisting arrest and assault on an officer.

When I heard this, I told him that my husband has a medical condition called Primary Progressive Aphasia and that he should have an identification tag around his neck.

The Officer said that he did not have anything on him and asked that I come to the hospital and we can talk some more.

I hung up the phone. Denise Banks, my co-worker, was standing near me and had heard my conversation with the officer.

I began to cry when I told her that Dan may be arrested for assaulting an officer and resisting arrest and she indicated that everything would be okay and that she would drive me to the hospital.

On the way to the hospital, I called Dan's brother Mike, who was a retired lieutenant with the Sheriff's Department. I told him what happened with Dan and wanted him to know what was going on in the event Dan got arrested.

Mike assured me that he didn't believe Dan would be arrested because of his medical condition and said to call him if I needed anything.

When I arrived at the hospital, we went to the emergency room and I asked to speak to Officer Gibson.

When Officer Gibson arrived a minute later, he explained to me what happened and that Dan was okay, just a little abrasion on his forehead, but that the doctor hadn't seen him yet so I had to wait in the waiting room.

Officer Gibson informed me that the car was impounded as well as the dog and that he would get the information as to where the car was taken and where the dog was taken so I could get them both out.

Denise was supportive and assured me that everything would be okay. She then drove me home to pick up the truck so that when Dan was released from the hospital, I could drive him home.

When I got home, I immediately went over to my neighbor's house to ask if they could take me to pick up the car from the impound lot. I told them the story about Dan. They were shocked and wanted to do whatever they could for me.

I drove back to the hospital and was able to see Dan.

When Dan first saw me his was so happy to see me and gave me a big kiss, and asked where the dog was. Dan then proceeded to tell me "that person did bad for me, I did everything perfect."

He then saw Officer Gibson standing a few feet away from him and said "that person took me down and he got the item from me." Which translates to: The Officer threw him to the ground and took his driver's license away.

Dan told the officer that he wanted his item back (meaning his driver's license) but the officer told him no, that "you did an error." Dan proceeded to raise his voice and said "No, you did an error for me; I did everything perfect."

I whispered in Officer Gibson's ear and asked him to tell Dan that everything was perfect so that Dan could calm down. The Officer told Dan, everything is okay and Dan finally calmed down. Dan then proceeded to tell me "The person did 10 items for me." I said "really."

I then asked Officer Gibson if he had called for back-up and he replied "Yes." I proceeded to tell Officer

Gibson that Dan said there were about 8 or 10 officers at the scene. Officer Gibson replied "that is about right."

While at home, I contacted Andrew Jared, the attorney at the office, and told him what the officer had said about the possibility of Dan being arrested for resisting arrest and assault on an officer.

Andrew said he would meet me at the hospital and would talk to Officer Gibson. While at the hospital Officer Gibson explained to me what had happened.

He said that he was at Azusa Canyon directing traffic and was only allowing residents into the canyon and that he had a section coned off. He said that Dan went around the cones and that's when he said "what's up with that person?"

He got in his squad car and followed Dan for about a mile with his siren on and speaker, asking Dan to pull over. Dan wouldn't pull over, but he was going the speed limit of 35 mph. The officer decided to pass Dan and cut him off to get him to stop.

Officer Gibson succeeded and when he got out of his vehicle, Dan shouted "that was bad, you did an error for me." This was the first clue there was something not right with Dan.

The officer asked Dan to turn off his engine, but Dan didn't understand his commands. The officer then grabbed Dan's hand and proceeded to shut the engine off. Then, he tried to get Dan to get out of the car, but

Dan refused. The officer then helped Dan remove the camera from around his neck and then when he did that, he proceeded to pull Dan out of the car, causing Dan to fall on top of him and onto the ground, wherein Dan scraped his head.

Once Officer Gibson got control of Dan, Dan was still non-responsive to his questioning. The officer noticed Dan had a wedding ring on and asked him what was the name of his wife so that he may contact her, but all Dan could say was he was doing 35 and that he did everything perfect and that he had to be somewhere.

At this point, several officers showed up (approx. 10) and one of them tried to talk to Dan, but Dan was not making any sense so Officer Gibson called for paramedics and Dan was taken to Foothill Presbyterian Hospital, which was located near our home.

Before Andrew arrived at the hospital, Officer Gibson informed me that he had spoken to his sergeant and explained Dan's medical condition. He requested that Dan be released to my custody. The sergeant said okay and that they would not be arresting him.

I was so relieved that they were not going to arrest Dan. Officer Gibson was apologetic for hurting Dan and I thanked him for recognizing that Dan had a medical condition and that Dan needed medical attention instead of beating him up and taking him to jail, or worse, be forced to use his weapon and kill Dan or wound him.

Had Dan gone to jail, that would have been a traumatic experience for him.

I explained to Officer Gibson that in Dan's mind, Dan wasn't doing anything wrong, that he was going the speed limit and was going to take the dog for a walk up at the canyon as he did every week.

Officer Gibson was very understanding and apologetic for hurting Dan and what he went through.

Andrew showed up at the hospital about 3:00 p.m. I introduced Officer Gibson to Andrew and said he was my attorney. Officer Gibson informed Andrew that they would be releasing Dan to my custody and that he would not be arrested, but that he would be making a report and it was up to the District Attorney's Office to press charges or not.

Officer Gibson didn't think they would but in any event, he still had to write his report. I thanked Andrew for coming to the hospital and for all his support.

I went back inside the emergency room where Dan was and told him everything was okay and that we would be going home soon. Dan said okay, let's order the dog. Dan was released to my custody at approximately 4:00 p.m.

We left the hospital, and I called my sister Margaret at work so that she could drive me to pick up the car and get the dog out of impound.

When I arrived at Margaret's work to pick her up, she was nervous and asked why I didn't call her sooner so that she could be with me. I said I was okay, that I didn't want to bother her at work.

We drove to Baldwin Park, which was approximately 15 to 20 minutes from Margaret's work. We were able to get the car out of impound just in time before they closed and we were able to pick up our dog Springer from the dog pound just before they closed too. Dan was so happy when we picked up Springer from the pound. This incident cost me $300.00 to get the car and the dog out of impound. That's cheap compared to what could have happened.

I had tickets for the Eagles concert that night at the Forum (floor seating) and I wanted to go and was also hoping that Dan would enjoy the concert and forget about what happened earlier in the day. Dan loves music, especially the Eagles. When we got to the Forum Dan had no clue who the Eagles were and had no interest in being there. All he wanted to do was go home. I said okay and we left the concert at around 10:30 p.m.

The following morning, Saturday, Dan was upset about the incident that had occurred yesterday and kept saying that the person did an error for him that he did everything perfect. I said okay Sweetiepie, let's go get something to eat and Dan said okay. We both got dressed and walked out the door and proceeded to walk down the street to a nearby restaurant.

As we walked down the street, there was a police patrol car around the corner from our house. Dan saw the vehicle and gave a direct stare at the officer seated inside the vehicle and proceeded to say "that person is bad, very bad, he did an error for me." I said it's okay Sweetiepie, let's go get something to eat. I thought to myself, how long will Dan believe that police officers are bad and how can I make him understand that they are here to protect us?

The following Tuesday January 27, 2014, I took the day off from work and took Dan to the DMV to get an identification card for him because Officer Gibson had taken his driver's license.

We arrived at the Rancho Cucamonga DMV office at 7:00 a.m., with the hopes that would be the first in line. Apparently everyone was thinking the same thing and there were at least 20 people ahead of us. We waited in line for an hour before they let us in. Dan didn't know why we were there and after an hour of waiting, Dan wanted to go home.

Dan doesn't understand that you have to sometimes wait hours at the DMV to get an Identification Card. While waiting the two hours to be seen, the DMV's computers shut down and we were told to come back tomorrow or make an appointment.

I said "no way, I can't do this again" so I walked up to the clerk and told her my situation. She told me to go to another DMV office and to tell the clerk that I have a disabled person, and that I would like a priority number, and that we should not have to wait too long.

I did what she told me and we went to another DMV near our home and it only took 30 minutes.

The following week, I wrote a letter to Captain S. Urrea of the California Highway Patrol and expressed my gratitude for Officer Gibson's actions and conduct that fateful day January 24, 2014.

A week later, I received a letter from Captain Urrea thanking me for my letter and indicating that he had shared my letter with Officer Gibson and the rest of his staff and was pleased to hear from me and hoped my husband was doing better.

Chapter 23

Court Appearance

Dan received a notice from the Court to appear on February 28, 2014 for the incident that occurred on January 24, 2014.

Charges were brought against him by the District Attorney's Office.   Dan was charged with assault on an officer, resisting arrest, and disobeying traffic signs.

I contacted Dan's doctor and explained Dan's situation and she requested I take Dan to get another PetScan.

In early February I took Dan to get another PetScan to see if his brain had changed from the prior scan taken in February 2010.

On February 20, 2014, we met with Dr. Chui to go over the results of the PetScan. Dan was happy to see the doctor because he thought he was going to see her so that he could get his license back. The doctor showed us the second PetScan and to my surprise, the disease had travelled to the right side of the brain.

The doctor later explained that the disease was already on the right side of the brain, just not moving as fast as the left.   This news was over whelming to me.   I didn't know what to expect for Dan's future after I received this information.   The doctor told Dan that this brain was having an error and showed Dan the image of his brain and that it travelled to the right side of his brain.

Dan understood what the doctor told him and he pointed to his head that it went from the left side to the right side. The doctor then told Dan that he could not drive the truck (order the truck because of the error in his brain). Dan didn't quite understand why he could not drive because in his mind, he did everything perfect.

Dan asked the doctor if they were going to fix the error in his brain and the doctor said we are trying to fix it and Dan replied, that's okay thank you very much. Dan then told the doctor he loved her and she replied, "I love you too."

We went downstairs to the lab where Dan gave a sample of his blood so that he could be in a study with other patients who had the same diagnosis. After we left the doctor's office, Dan indicated to me that in 2011 they did not take blood from him, and I said you're right, they did not take blood from you the last time. I love you, let's go home.

Dr. Chui wrote a letter to the Court on Dan's behalf explaining Dan's diagnosis and that his condition had progressed to the extent that she felt Dan's driving privileges should be revoked.

I was nervous for Dan because I did not know how he was going to react in court.

You see, after the incident that took place on January 24, 2014, Dan has a different opinion of police officers. He believes they are bad people. Even though Dan's brother Mike is a retired lieutenant with and his nephew Shane is a deputy with the Sheriff's Department, Dan still believes they are bad people.

Due to Dan's medical condition, he cannot comprehend why the officer pulled him over and forcefully pulled him out of his vehicle and arrested him.

I was fortunate enough to work for a law firm that is familiar with criminal law, not to mention to be employed by a very dear friend of mine, Roger, who agreed to represent Dan in court for free. I explained to him all about Dan's medical condition and he assured me that Dan would not be charged with any crime.

We appeared in court on February 28, 2014. I was still very nervous, not because I was afraid that the charges against Dan would stick, but because I wasn't sure how Dan was going to react in court.

We arrived at court at 7:30 a.m. and waited in line outside the courthouse until the doors opened at 8:00 a.m. Dan had no idea why we were at that location so early in the morning. But when we got inside, somehow Dan believed we were there to get his driver's license back because he asked if we were there for him. I said yes, we are here for you.

Roger appeared at 8:30 a.m., I introduced Roger to Dan and Dan shook his hand and had a smile on his face and asked Roger if he was here for him. Roger said yes, everything is going to be okay.

We waited outside the courtroom until 9:00 a.m. until the doors to the courtroom opened. We sat in the front row of the courtroom while Roger went to see if he could find the district attorney who would be appearing.

A few minutes later, Roger appeared and said he was unable to talk to the attorney who would be appearing.

Dan asked if Roger was going to get it for him and I said "Yes, he is going to help you, just lower your voice and wait for Roger to call us, okay."

A half hour later, the attorney appeared and Roger sat next to her and was speaking to her before the judge appeared on the bench.

A few minutes later, they called Dan's name and Roger and the attorney appeared before the court. The district attorney informed the court that she needed a continuance on the matter because she just got back from vacation and had not had enough time to review the case.

Roger agreed to the continuance and the matter was continued for another week.

I was hoping it would be all over, but I understood. We were prepared and I was able to get a letter from Dan's neurologist informing the court about Dan's medical condition. It stated that Dan was unaware of what was happening around him and that Dan's Aphasia had progressed to thc cxtcnt that shc fclt his driving privileges should be taken away.

We left the courtroom and Dan again asked if we were there for him so that he could get his driver's license back. How Dan knew this, I will never know.

It is now March 5, 2014, our return court date. I was not as nervous as before but just the same, I wanted all three charges against Dan to be dismissed.

Roger explained to me that it was a good possibility that two of the three charges would be dropped, but that the traffic violation (the most minor of the three charges) would not be dropped. I said "okay, I understand."

The hearing took only 10 minutes. Roger and the attorney approached the bench and explained to the judge Dan's medical condition and that they had agreed to dismiss 2 of the 3 counts against Dan.

The judge then called Dan's name and Dan and I approached the court. It was quick, and the judge said that Dan would be charged with vehicle code 21461(A) and was ordered to pay a fine of $350.00.

Dan's driver's license would also be revoked and the deputy sitting to our right approached Dan and handed him a notice of revoked driver's license form which Dan had to sign. A minute later the court dismissed us and we were free to go.

The Truck Taken away from Dan

After the January 24th incident, Dan was no longer able to drive. He had a difficult time accepting that he could not drive. He would say that he paid for the two cars in the driveway and he should be able to drive them. I tried to explain to Dan that his brain is having an error and that's why he can't drive. His reply was that he does everything perfect and that he should be able to use the two items (cars).

It's been 3 months now since Dan has driven. At least I thought he was not driving until my neighbor Wendy called me at work April 24th to say that she saw Dan drive in our driveway. I said "thank you" and raced home from work to get the keys away from him. When I got home I asked Dan if he drove the truck and

he said "no I did not." I told him that is not the truth, that he drove the truck and I want the keys back right now. Dan denied taking the truck and only after I told him that I was leaving did he finally hand me the keys.

I tried to explain to Dan that he is having an error in his brain and that's why he cannot drive the truck. He says "okay" and I placed the keys in my purse.

Two weeks later, I was getting ready for work and checked my purse to make sure the keys were there. When I saw that they were missing, I asked Dan where the key to the truck was and he denied having the key.

I told him he had it and I wanted it immediately. He again said he did not have it so I walked away from him and seconds later he handed the keys to me, says that I placed the keys in the bedroom, and that he found the key.

This happened again the following week so now I have to hide the key somewhere other than in my purse because I cannot trust Dan anymore.

It's now June, six months later and Dan has finally accepted the fact that he cannot drive. What a relief!

Chapter 24

My Most Challenging Event

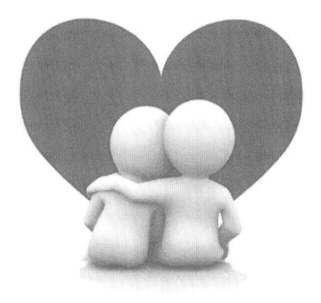

The most challenging thing for me was trying to get the financial assistance I needed to help with Dan's homecare. We didn't have long-term medical care to help with the future care Dan would need when his condition progressed.

Because our monthly income exceeded the required state and VA guidelines we were not eligible for any government assistance to help with Dan's homecare.

We have to pay out-of-pocket for homecare expenses which average $720.00 a month. You either have to be very poor or extremely rich to get the help you need from the government.

Then it was trying to find someone who I trusted to care for Dan and who understood his condition and who Dan could feel comfortable with. It's not easy finding someone who you trust. You hear about so many elderly men and women and young children being abused while in the care of their caregivers. I didn't want that to happen to Dan so I had to find someone who was reliable and who I trusted.

Then I remembered that my friend Marichelle's step-son, Shane, lived in Glendora, just 2 miles away from our home, and he and Dan knew each other. So in February of 2014, I hired him to stay with Dan a couple of hours a day so that Dan wouldn't be home alone all day while I worked and would make sure Dan had something to eat.

The first two weeks Dan wasn't sure why Shane was coming over every day. Dan knew Shane was related to Marichelle, but he still didn't trust him.

By the 3rd week, Dan became more comfortable with Shane and began to trust him and things were working out great. Shane was a college student and had another part-time job so sometimes he was unable to stay with Dan.

I understood, but at the same time, I worried that Dan was home alone and had no one to talk to and would have to ride his bicycle to go get something to eat. I would buy frozen dinners for him to eat at lunch time and warm up in the microwave but often times Dan wouldn't eat them.

Dan was not allowed to use the oven because one day, I came home from work and the house smelled of gas.

I immediately went to the kitchen to see if one of the pilot lights was on and sure enough, Dan had not shut the burner off correctly. Thank God, Dan didn't light a match or caused something to spark, otherwise the house and Dan would have gone up in smoke.

After this incident, I made sure Dan didn't cook anything in the house and made sure someone was with him during the lunch hour to take him out to lunch or warm up the food I had left in the refrigerator for him.

Shane was wonderful, he would take Dan to the arboretum and out to get something to eat, and sometimes he would bring Dan to my work so that we could have lunch together, which Dan really enjoyed.

This worked out great for about six months, and then Shane was working more hours at his part-time job and was only able to stay with Dan two days a week, which meant Dan had to ride his bicycle to get something to eat on the days that Shane couldn't make it. This made me nervous, because Dan has no sense of danger and I was afraid that Dan would get hit by a car.

One day, when I got home from work, I noticed Dan had a large wound on his right arm. I pointed to his arm and asked what happened. Because Dan is unable to communicate, he motioned that he fell off his bike. It was a pretty bad road burn. He had taken the third layer of skin off his arm. Dan said he was alright and didn't want medical attention. I cleaned the wound and kept it bandaged for a couple of days.

When it didn't look like it was healing, I took Dan to the urgent care facility to have it looked at. Just getting Dan to see the doctor was a challenge. Dan didn't want to see the doctor, he said he was fine. I finally got Dan to go to the doctor.

The doctor who examined Dan said he had a third degree burn on his arm and that those take longer to heal and to just keep an eye on it in the event of infection.

After this incident, I was determined to find someone to help me with Dan so I began to search again on the internet and made several calls to different government agencies, but to no avail.

I had to do something, so I spoke to my office manager and explained the situation I was having with Dan.

My AGC family have been so understanding about Dan's medical condition, they agreed to allow me to reduce my hours so that I could be home with Dan at 1:30 p.m. on Tuesdays and Thursdays. Now I had to find someone to stay with Dan on Mondays, Wednesdays and Fridays on a permanent basis.

Then, one day, while I was talking to my niece Bertha, who happens to live 9 miles away from our home, I told her my situation and asked if she knew anyone who could help me with Dan, who was honest and reliable.

She indicated that she could stay with Dan on those days. I said really, I thought you were taking care of your two nephews for your sister. She indicated that they were starting preschool in August and that she would be available on those days. I was so relieved that she would be able to stay with Dan.

Shane was working more hours for his other employer and was not available half the time I needed him so I told Shane that I needed someone on a permanent basis. Shane understood my situation and thanked me for giving him a job and I thanked him for all his help with Dan.

Since Bertha has been staying with Dan, he seems to be a lot happier and is trying to talk more. I have to pay out-of-pocket, but it's worth every penny to come home and find Dan is happy and healthy. I no longer have to worry that he will get hurt while riding his bicycle.

That has to be the most challenging thing for me, finding someone who you trust who could take care of the one you love and make sure he is happy.

Chapter 25

Another Step in Dan's Condition

Dan's condition is progressive and mimics many of the same characteristics of Alzheimer's disease, one of which is agoraphobia (ag-uh-ruh-FOE-be-uh), a type of anxiety disorder in which you fear and often avoid places or situations that might cause you to panic and make you feel trapped, helpless, or embarrassed.

With agoraphobia, you fear an actual or anticipated situation, such as using public transportation, being in open or enclosed spaces, standing in line or being in a crowd. The anxiety is caused by fear that there's no easy way to escape or seek help if intense anxiety develops. Most people who have agoraphobia develop it after having one or more panic attacks, causing them to fear another attack and avoid the place where it occurred.

People with agoraphobia often have a hard time feeling safe in any public place, especially where crowds gather. You may feel that you need a companion, such as a relative or friend, to go with you to public places. The fears can be so overwhelming that you may feel unable to leave your home.

Agoraphobia treatment can be challenging because it usually means confronting your fears. But with talk therapy (psychotherapy) and medications, you can escape the trap of agoraphobia and live a more enjoyable life.

November 12, 2014, we were packed and out the door by 9:00 a.m. The temperature was 54 degrees in Glendora on this sunny Wednesday morning, when we headed for Scottsdale, Arizona to stay with our cousin

Maria and Lou for the night before driving to Prescott, Arizona to visit Dan's daughter Maureen, grandson Gino and newly born granddaughter, Ember Rose. I was well rested for the 5 ½ hour drive.

A few minutes into our drive, Dan said he wanted to get something to eat so I exited the freeway on Foothill Boulevard and stopped at Starbucks to get him something to eat.

As we entered Starbucks, I asked Dan what he wanted to eat, he pointed at the croissant and then said he was having an error and pointed to his stomach and he needed to go to the bathroom. I waited for Dan to get out of the bathroom. When he exited the bathroom, he didn't look good. He had just thrown up and wanted to sit down. I helped him sit down in a chair and asked the clerk for some water to give him.

Dan then said that he had did 4 times. I said "what did you do 4 times?"

He again replied, "I did it for 4 times." I wasn't sure what he was saying, did he threw up or did he go to the bathroom 4 times? I couldn't make out what he was trying to say. I then said "do you still want to eat" and he replied "No, he wanted out" which was to go in the car.

We sat inside Starbucks for about 10 minutes and then we got up and Dan walked to the car without any problem. I again asked "are you okay?" He said "temporarily." I thought to myself, maybe he ate something that didn't agree with him and that he would be okay. We got on the 210 Freeway headed east.

A few minutes later, Dan was uncomfortable in the front seat, so I exited the freeway again so that he could lie down in the back seat of the car. It was now 10:00 a.m. and we had only driven 15 miles from our home. Dan said no, that he wanted to sit in the front seat, and wanted me to put back the head rest that I had taken off earlier so that he could rest better with a head pillow.

When we got to Palm Desert, which was about an hour and a half away from home, I pulled off to get gas. I asked Dan if he wanted to lie down in the back seat of the car. Dan said yes, temporarily. I got him some Sprite® which he drank and then curled up in the back seat of the car with a blanket that I brought along for the ride.

I entered the freeway again and said a prayer that we would make it safely to the Arizona state line where I could gas up again. Dan slept the entire 3 hour trip until we got to the Arizona border. Dan woke up and asked that I get him a Coke®, I said okay, "do you want to stay in the car or do you want to get off?"

He said he wanted to get off so we both walked into the store and I bought him his Coke®. I asked if he was hungry and he said no. I filled up the tank and headed east again. Dan was now in the front seat of the car.

A half hour into the drive, Dan began to shake his arms uncontrollably, he looked pale white and his hands and arm felt clammy to the touch. His eyes began to roll back as he proceeded to put his head down. I tried talking to him but he was non-responsive.

I immediately called 911 and in a soft and calm voice, informed the operator that my husband did not look well, that he was shaking uncontrollably for approximately 5 seconds or so and was non-responsive and that he looked pale white, and that he had no color to his face.

The operator asked where I was, I told her that we had just passed the Wickenberg/Parker exit and that we were about 2 miles east on the 10 Freeway.

She asked if I had pulled over to the side of the road and I said no not yet. She instructed me to pull over and that she would call for paramedics to my location shortly.

I said okay and pulled over.

She then asked how Dan was doing, and I said that he was no longer shaking, but that he did not look good.

She asked if he had any medical condition and I said yes, he has a medical condition called Primary Progressive Aphasia but that otherwise, he was in perfect health. She said okay thank you, help should be on the way shortly and then hung up.

After about 5 minutes or so of trying to get my husband's attention he decided to get out of the car, I said "no, stay in the car." He refused and then proceeded to open the door. I immediately jumped out of the car and walked around towards the passenger's side of the car. Dan wanted to lie down in the back of the car and I assisted him and he just laid there curled up. I tried to get him to sip a cup of water, but he refused.

I still can't believe how calm I was about what just happened. As I sat in the car waiting for help to arrive, I couldn't help but think, of all places for Dan to get sick it would have to be in the middle of nowhere on Highway 10.

I said to myself, "who can I call and talk to while I'm waiting for help to arrive?" I immediately thought of Rachel; she will understand and not panic.

I called Rachel and told her what happened to Dan. She immediately said she thought he may have food poisoning and that he was dehydrated and that's why he was clammy to the touch and pale white. She also lectured me about driving to Arizona when Dan didn't feel well. I told her that I thought he would sleep it off and would feel better once he got some rest. She assured me that he would be okay and we talked until the Highway Patrol officer arrived.

When the Officer Schmitt arrived I told him that I thought Dan may have food poisoning and was probably dehydrated but that I was not sure. A few minutes later, the paramedics arrived and hooked Dan up to a monitor to check his vitals. Dan was non-coherent and just laid in the back of the car seat.

I explained to the paramedic that Dan had a medical condition call Primary Progressive Aphasia and that he is unable to communicate and tell me what's wrong with him, but that he had mentioned earlier that he had done something 4 times but I wasn't sure what he was talking about at the time, but that now that I think about it, he had probably thrown up or went to the bathroom 4 times and that would explain why he was not feeling well.

The paramedic evaluating Dan printed out a report and he indicated that Dan did not have a seizure or a stroke and that he was probably dehydrated and that his condition was not life threatening, but if I wanted them to take him to the hospital that the closest hospital was 60 miles away. I told him no, if his condition was not life threatening, that I would drive to Scottsdale and if his condition worsened, that I would stop at the nearest emergency room.

He said okay and then had me sign a release for non-medical treatment. I thanked him and the officer for their time and assistance and drove away.

I finally made it to Scottsdale, Arizona. It was 6:30 p.m. when we arrived at my cousin's house. I got out of the car and helped Dan inside the house. Dan did not know where we were and I asked my cousin Marina to give Dan a glass of Gatorade®. Dan drank the Gatorade and asked if he could lie down. I walked him to the bedroom and helped him to the bed.

Dan slept all through the night and woke up around 5:00 a.m. asking to go home to our dogs. I told him we would go home on Sunday, but he didn't understand. I said to go back to sleep and that we would get up at 8:00 a.m.

When we finally woke up, Dan wanted to go to the bathroom, I assisted him to the bathroom and as he took his pants off, I saw that he had pooped on his shorts. I tried to get him to take them off, but he refused. I finally convinced him that if he took them off we could go home, but that he needed to take a shower first. He said okay and I assisted him into the shower. I stayed in the bathroom while he showered in the event he fell or needed help getting out of the tub.

He did not look well; he had gotten some color back, but still looked pale. I gave him some clean clothes and help dress him and went into the living room to where my cousin Marina and her husband Lou were.

She asked Dan how he was feeling and Dan didn't respond. She asked Dan if he wanted to eat and Dan said no. She then handed Dan a glass of Gatorade® and told him to drink it that he would feel better.

Dan wanted to go home to his dogs and I said we were going to see his daughter Maureen and Gino, but Dan didn't understand. A half hour later, I was ready to go. I don't think Dan knew where we were and kept saying he wanted to go home to his dogs.

I thanked my cousin for a good night's rest and then went on our way to Prescott. Dan was somewhat alert, but still had no idea where we were. When we arrived at his daughter's house, he did not want to go in.

I said "it's your daughter Maureen's house" but there was still no response from him. His daughter opened the door and greeted him, but there was still no reaction from him. We went inside the house and he did not recognize his daughter or his grandson. I believe in his mind that these were people I knew and we were only their visiting for a short time.

He didn't talk much, just asked how old the new baby was and Maureen said 5 weeks and he replied "oh really." He then sat on the couch and I gave him something to drink. He just sat on the couch not saying anything.

Maureen made Dan and I a grilled cheese sandwich of which he ate only half and a few minutes later, he asked to go to the bathroom. When he didn't come out, I went to see what he was doing and I found him asleep in the bedroom.

An hour later, Dan woke up in a better mood, I'm not sure if he was aware that we were at his daughter's home. I took lots of pictures of him and the kids before we went for a walk to downtown Prescott for some fresh air. Dan still didn't recognize that we were in Prescott, Arizona.

When we got back to Maureen's place, Dan wanted to go home. I told him okay, we will go to the room in

197

our hotel. We said goodbye and headed for the hotel, which was about 2 miles away.

We checked into the hotel and rested before going back to Maureen's for dinner later that evening.

When we got to Maureen's house Dan didn't want to get out of the car. I said "we are going to eat, come on let's go." He finally got out of the car and went inside.

Dan still had no clue where we were.
We sat and ate dinner and I made small talk while Dan just sat on the couch.

We finally left around 8:00 pm to head back to the hotel. Dan again said he wanted to go home, I said "okay, tomorrow we will go home" and he said "okay."

The next morning, we went to Maureen's home for breakfast and Dan still had no idea where we were.

We all then got in the car and went to Ross Department store for some shopping. Dan got out of the car, but then a few minutes later wanted to go sit in the car. I said okay, we will be there soon. A half hour or so later, Dan came back into the store looking for me. He said he wanted to go home. I said okay, let's go. We all got in the car and headed back to Maureen's place. I dropped off Maureen and the kids and Dan and I went back to the hotel.

When we got to the hotel, Dan motioned to go to the registration desk to check out. I said no, we have to go upstairs first. When we got to our room, I told Dan to lie down for a while. He said no, that he wanted to go home and proceeded to get our bags. I said okay, let's go home. He said okay.

We checked out and I headed back to Maureen's place to say goodbye. Dan refused to get out of the car and I had to ask Maureen to see if she could get him to get out of the car. She told him she wanted him to take some pictures of her and the kids and then he finally got out of the car.

I took some pictures of Dan, Maureen, and the kids, and told Maureen that we had to leave because her dad wanted to go home and I didn't want to force him to stay. She understood, but had tears in her eyes because we were leaving and she didn't have enough time to spend with her dad. I told her I was sorry again, but I had to do what was best for her dad, and right now, he wants to go home.

As we were getting in the car and saying our goodbyes, Dan finally recognized where we were and said he had been there before and I said yes, we were here before a year ago. I think he was finally realizing that we were in Prescott, Arizona visiting his daughter. He gave his daughter a hug and a kiss and we got in the car and headed back to Scottsdale, to stay at my cousin's house before going home.

When we got to my cousin's house, Dan recognized the house this time and when he saw my cousin Lou, he recognized him too and said he had been there before and that Lou had 3 items (which meant, this was a 3 bedroom house) and I said "yes, Sweetiepie, this has 3 items."

Dan was hungry and wanted to get something to eat, so I ordered a hamburger from a nearby restaurant and then he and Lou went to pick it up. Dan was so happy when he got his hamburger and fries, and was excited that the young girls gave him a coke. Dan ate his hamburger and was in a better mood and even got some color back in his face.

When my cousin arrived later that evening from work, Dan recognized her too and later made small talk with her about his brain having an error, that was his own way of apologizing for not being able to communicate with her. My cousin said that's okay and then he told her "I love you."

We both went to bed around 9 p.m. and were up by 7:00 a.m. I wanted to get an early start back home. Dan was dressed and ready to go by 7:30 a.m. He was so happy we were going home.

As we drove away, Dan was directing me where to go.

I was surprised he knew the way back to the freeway, considering he was asleep when we arrived on Wednesday night.

As I entered the 101 west Freeway, Dan said I was going the wrong way and that I had to go east. I said no, we have to go west and Dan insisted that we go east.

As I continued West on the 101 Dan began to get nervous and had tears in his eyes and said I was doing bad. I said "no Sweetiepie, we are okay, we have to go west" and he again said no, we have to back. I tried to assure him that we were okay.

As we entered the 10 Freeway West, Dan began to panic and looked scared. I tried to calm him down and say that we were going home to the dogs, but he was sure I was going the wrong way. I just kept talking to him the entire drive home, telling him that we would see Springer, Sportster, and ChuChu at home. Dan still had tears in his eyes and looked scared. I said "it's okay, we are going home."

When we made it to the California state line, Dan felt a little better. We stopped and bought gas and I assured Dan that we would be home in 3 hours. We got back in the car and headed west.

When Dan saw the sign that read "210 Pasadena," he was so excited that we were almost home and said that I did perfect. I said "I know Sweetiepie, we are almost home," and then he replied, "You're great, you are doing great."

I believe this was the beginning of Dan's agoraphobia.

You never know when your loved one will develop this condition, until it happens. There is no way to predict it either, because unless your loved one begins to panic as you leave the home, you have no idea what's up ahead until it happens. It's a live and learn situation. There is no book that can prepare you for life's lessons.

What I can tell you from my experience is once your loved one can no longer work, he should not be left alone for long periods of time. As I found out from leaving Dan alone while I worked to provide for our family, his ability to communicate with me and others deteriorated quickly because he didn't have anyone to talk to during the day.

I thought that because his condition was progressing, that his ability to communicate with me and others would cease as well. That is not true. The only reason (I believe) his ability to communicate with me decreased more quickly was because he didn't have anyone to talk to during the day. It wasn't until my sister and her daughter moved in with us for 3 months, that Dan began to communicate more. When they moved out Dan's ability to communicate with me and others slowly stopped.

Keeping active and having some type of communication with your loved one on a daily basis can help with the progression.

I know this for a fact, because since my niece Bertha has been staying with him three hours a day for the past seven months, Dan is a lot happier and although he cannot say the words he wants to stay, he sure tries to communicate with me and others.

Bertha also works with him during the day and shows him pictures of family and friends and also shows him flash cards of various items around the house and pictures. Dan can remember some of them, when he is trying to communicate with me.

Chapter 26

Where I'm At Now That I Understand What's Happening

Now that I know what's happening with Dan, I see things more clearly and I have learned to have more patience with him.

I don't yell anymore when he doesn't understand or listen to what I am asking him to do.

We have developed a new way of communicating. Dan has a limited vocabulary and depending on where we are, like inside the house, outside, at a restaurant, or at the doctor's office, I know how to figure out exactly what he wants.

It's like having a child that is learning how to talk and they have their own language and you start to pick up their language and repeat what they say and it works.

We are so much in love with each other now more than ever because I understand Dan. Dan knows he has a problem with his brain which limits is ability to talk and do things. We are so much happier and I thank God every day that I was given the love of my life back. Accepting and understanding what Primary Progressive Aphasia is all about is a first step in moving forward to a healthier and loving relationship.

I'm not saying that it is going to get easier, in fact, it may get harder at times. But, how you handle each situation that you come across and learn what works and what doesn't work makes your life a lot easier.

Nothing happens overnight, it takes time, love, and compassion to overcome any obstacle that you face.

You also have to remember that you need to take care of yourself and not only your loved one.

Take time for yourself and go shopping, get your nails done, have lunch or dinner with friends. Do whatever makes you happy for a couple of hours. If it means hiring someone to stay with your loved one for a couple of hours, do it.

You need to find time to exercise too to release the tension you sometimes get with working and caring for your loved one.

My worry now is that I may die before Dan because of the stress associated with his condition, and that no one would be able to care for Dan the way I do.

Because of the progression of the disease, Dan's condition can change year to year and the changes are gradual, not all of a sudden.

It is sometimes difficult to make his life as simple and happy as possible because Dan doesn't always understand what I am saying or why I'm doing the things that I am doing. We visit his mother and father often, which makes Dan very happy.

Dan's brother, Mike, has been spending more time with Dan and visits him regularly.

They go out to lunch and Dan directs Mike where to go to get something to eat. Mike is starting to get to know Dan's language and he enjoys seeing a smile on his brother's face when he comes to visit. I know that

Dan looks forward to seeing his brother. I am grateful that Mike is spending time with his brother and that they understand one another. I can see the love that they have for one another when I see them together.

I am so grateful that we were given a second chance to fall in love again and begin a new chapter in our lives together.

Chapter 27

Implementing Coping Mechanisms That Work

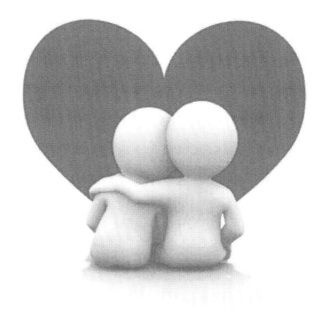

When I first learned of Dan's condition, I wasn't sure how we would communicate with one another. But what I did know was that Dan was good with numbers so I had to figure out how I could use numbers to replace words.

For instance, when I wanted to have sex I would often ask Dan if he wanted to have fun.

Dan would often confuse "do you want to have fun" with going out and doing something fun to do. So one day, while we were in bed, I had asked Dan if he wanted to have fun and Dan said no thank you.

Then one evening, while we were in bed, I said to Dan, (while touching his penis), Sweetiepie, if I want to have sex, I am going to say "do you want to have number 3."

Dan said okay. I wasn't sure if Dan understood what I meant, but later that evening about 1:30 a.m., I placed my hand on his penis and began to stroke it and Dan replied, "No Sweetiepie, let's do number 3 in the morning." I was amazed that he understood what I said earlier that evening.

After that, whenever either one of us wanted to have sex, we would say "do you want to do number 3." We were both happy that we had a new code word for "sex."

We developed a number system that worked whenever Dan wanted to get something to eat or go to the bathroom or when he wanted to take the dogs for a walk. The number system worked for about 2 years and then Dan forgot about number 3.

Now if we are out shopping or at a friend or families home, Dan will look around for the bathroom, and I somehow know what he wants and I direct him to the bathroom.

When I have trouble understanding what Dan is trying to say, I grab his hand and tell him to show me. I tell him I don't understand, and he will try and tell me again what he wants.

Sometimes, I have to get the keys to the car and show him if he wants me to drive him somewhere. If he wants me to take him somewhere, he will direct me where to go.

He sometimes uses the word "the big item," which could mean a number of things, depending on what has occurred during the day or where we are.

Ordering food at a restaurant is pretty easy for Dan; he just looks at the pictures displayed on the board and says the number of the item he wants. However, when he looks at a menu, he is unable to choose what he wants, unless he sees the words "Burger/Chicken," then he will point to that, otherwise, I will order for him. It is good to know what the other person likes to cat so you can order for them.

We try to have a daily routine, so that Dan knows what's going on around him. If I'm going to be late from work, I will let Dan know ahead of time. Since

Dan is good with numbers, I will say "I will order for you at 1:30; 6:30; 8:00 or 9:00 and Dan understands. If someone will be coming over to stay with him, I will show him the pictures of the person coming over and will tell him that "the person will order for you at 11:00."

When Dan was in Speech Therapy, the therapist made him a book with pictures of friends, family members, our dogs, and other items around the house to help Dan remember their names. This was and is a big help. We continue to add pictures in the book and go over the book with Dan at least 2 or 3 times a week.

Another mechanism that works is if you look at that person in the eyes and get their attention and speak to them slowly. If you talk too fast, they cannot understand what you are saying. Do not raise your voice and yell at them, they cannot function if you yell at them.

Marking the calendar of events that are coming-up is helpful too. This will give the person something to look forward to.

If we are going somewhere and will be gone for several hours, don't tell the person the exact time you will return, tell them at least 1 hour ahead of the time you expect to be home. (For example, if you want to be home by 3:00 o'clock, say you will be home at 4:00 o'clock), otherwise, they will bug you if you do not leave on time, that way if you leave an hour before the time you told them, they will be happy and not get anxious about coming home late.

Other coping and support mechanisms that help would be to pay close attention to the affected person, providing more time for communication, keep statements short and brief and supplementing speech with gestures.

If we are going out to a special event, I set out his clothes on the bed and show him that I want him to wear that item. Often times, Dan will wear a pair of jeans and t-shirt and a cap on his head and will put the wrong pair of shoes on or sometimes he will wear the same clothes for 2 or 3 days. I have to tell him to change his clothes because they are dirty and sometimes I have to tell him to take a bath.

I feel like I have a child and often treat him like a child, which my friends and family tell me I should treat him like an adult. I often give in to his demands, only because I don't want to get into an argument with him, which sometimes causes Dan to get angry and throw things or hit the nearest object closest to him.

This is something I am definitely working on.

Ernestina Connolly

Chapter 28

A Physician's Perspective

Just to be sure that this is a clinically accurate representation of the stories and experiences that I've written about, I asked Dr. Chui, Dan's physician to answer some questions about the condition, its current status, and what we can expect in the future.

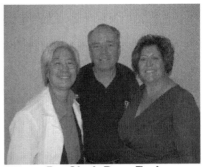

Dr. Chui, Dan, Erni

What is the exact name of Dan's condition?

It's called Primary Progressive Aphasia (PPA)

What does that mean in layman's language?

Aphasia is the loss of ability to understand or express language (spoken or written), caused by brain damage.

People with primary progressive aphasia have trouble expressing their thoughts and comprehending or finding words. The pattern of symptoms in PPA differs from the most common forms of dementia (such as Alzheimer disease) that begin with recent memory loss.

The most common cause of aphasia is a stroke. On the other hand, PPA is a rare nervous system (neurological) syndrome that is caused by a neurodegenerative disease, rather than stroke.

Neurodegenerative diseases are a group of disorders that cause slowly progressive loss of neurological function. These include Alzheimer disease (AD), Parkinson disease (PD), and amyotrophic lateral sclerosis (ALS).

Abnormal changes start at the molecular and microscopic level affecting the internal function within nerve cells and the electrical connections (synapses) between nerve cells.

Eventually, nerve cells shrink and die, which becomes manifest as progressive atrophy of the brain on neuroimaging studies (CAT or MRI scans).

The molecular changes responsible for neurodegeneration are not fully understood. Misfolded proteins appear to be a common thread. PPA has been associated with abnormal forms of several proteins, including tau, TDP-43, and progranulin.

How common is it?

The exact numbers are unknown because for many people it tends to mimic dementia and, if the patient is elderly, is treated exactly the same way without anyone knowing the specific cause of the condition.

How is it contracted?

Once again, the specifics are unknown and although there have been suspicions that have become the seminal points for ongoing research; there is currently no absolute evidence as to its origins or causes.

Is it hereditary?

As above, it's a possible cause but the current data and research does not support any definitive conclusions.

Some forms of PPA are hereditary and passed from one generation to the next. Others result from de novo changes in the genes. Some may be related to interactions between genes and environmental exposures.

What are the symptoms?

This type of aphasia begins gradually, with speech or language symptoms that will vary depending on the brain areas affected by the disease.

For example, in one type of PPA, people may initially have trouble producing speech, or articulating, whereas in another variant, word-finding and comprehension problems are more pronounced.

The majority of patients with PPA have problems expressing themselves with language while memory stays relatively intact, especially during the first two years of decline.

How does the condition progress in terms of physical and mental limitations or impairments?

Symptoms of primary progressive aphasia begin gradually, sometimes before age 65, and tend to worsen over time. People with primary progressive aphasia can become mute and may eventually lose the ability to understand written or spoken language.

People with primary progressive aphasia may continue caring for themselves and participating in daily life activities for several years after the disorder's onset, as the condition progresses slowly.

Is there a cure for it?

Not at the present time although there is ongoing research being conducted.

Does the condition get progressively worse?

Regrettably, yes. Since it may progress from aphasia to a more generalized form of dementia it's likely that the patent will slip into the same degenerative characteristics as an Alzheimer's patent which will eventually result in death.

Is the condition reversible?

Not at the present time. There is ongoing research into brain functions but there is no cure or reversing treatment at this time.

What research is being done to find a cure?

Multidisciplinary research is currently being conducted toward the treatment and cure of neurological diseases affecting cognition–focused on memory, language, and attention, auditory, visual and thinking difficulties.

These research programs and clinical care centers are devoted to the prevention, treatment and cure of Alzheimer's disease, Lewy body dementia, prion diseases, vascular dementia, traumatic brain injury, frontotemporal dementia, hydrocephalus, and autism.

How is it diagnosed?

A thorough evaluation of PPA includes the following:

- **History:** First, a careful history is taken to establish that a condition of dementia exists. This often requires that family members or friends be questioned about the patient's behavior because sometimes the patient is unaware of the symptoms (as in the case of memory loss or personality changes) or may be unable to describe them due to aphasia.

- **Neurological Examination:** A neurological examination is done to determine if there are signs of dementia on a simple screening of mental functions (the mental status examination) and also if there are signs of motor or sensory symptoms that indicate other types of neurological disorders might be causing the dementia. The neurologist will also order tests (e.g., blood tests, spinal tap, brain imaging studies) to further investigate the cause of the symptoms.

- **Neuropsychological Examination:** A neuropsychological examination provides a more detailed evaluation of mental functioning. This is especially important in the very early stages of illness when a routine screening evaluation may not detect the problems the patient is experiencing. This requires several hours and consists of paper-and-pencil or computer-administered tests of mental abilities, including attention and concentration, language, learning and memory, visual perception, reasoning and mood. The results can indicate if there are abnormalities of thinking and behavior and also their degree–mild, moderate or severe. It is often difficult to demonstrate that individuals with PPA have intact memory since we usually test memory by telling a person some information and then asking them to repeat it later on. In an individual with PPA, it may be impossible to repeat back the information because of the aphasia. Therefore, it is important that testing is done properly to make sure that there is not a true loss of memory.

- **Speech and Language Evaluation:** Since a decline in language abilities is the primary symptom of PPA, it is important to determine which components of language use are most affected, how severely affected they are, and what can be done to improve communication. A Speech-Language Pathologist evaluates different aspects of language in detail and can make recommendations for strategies to improve communication. Family members should be included in the treatment sessions to educate them about how to facilitate communication.

- **Psychosocial Evaluation:** PPA affects not only the individual who is suffering from this disorder, but also all people who are close to the patient. The disorder has an impact on relationships, the ability to continue working, the ability to perform many routine duties, and the ability to communicate even the simplest of needs. Although there are many resources available for individuals with memory loss, there are relatively fewer appropriate resources for individuals with PPA, their relatives and friends. Evaluation with a social worker who is familiar with PPA can address these issues and provide suggestions for dealing with day-to-day frustrations and problems.

- **Brain Imaging Studies:** The evaluation for dementia also includes a brain imaging study. This is done in the form of a computed axial tomography scan (CAT scan) or a magnetic resonance imaging scan (MRI scan). Both of these methods provide a picture of the brain so that any structural abnormalities, such as a stroke, tumor or hydrocephalus–all of which can give rise to dementia-like symptoms, can be detected. In the case of degenerative brain disease, the CAT scan and MRI scan may show "atrophy," which suggests "shrinkage" of the brain tissue. However, especially in early stages, they may not show anything. In fact, the report often comes back "normal." But this only means that there is no evidence for a tumor or stroke. It cannot tell us anything about the microscopic degenerative changes that have occurred.

- **Psychiatric Evaluation:** Sometimes there will also be a need for a psychiatric evaluation. This may be the case when it is not clear if the changes in behavior are due to depression or another psychiatric disturbance. Also, some individuals, especially those with PPA, may become saddened by their condition and may require treatment for depression.

- There are many thousands of people with PPA. Nonetheless, compared to the millions of patients with Alzheimer-type amnestic dementias, PPA is rare. Furthermore, it can start in a person's 40s and 50s, an age range that physicians do not usually associate with neurodegenerative diseases. Therefore, some people with PPA often see multiple doctors and receive many different diagnoses before receiving the diagnosis of PPA.

What is the treatment?

People with language difficulties may benefit from speech therapy to help them learn alternative ways to supplement and compensate for their lost skills. Maintaining adequate communication and social connections is critical.

Unlike many people who develop aphasia from head injury or stroke, people with PPA do not typically improve with time, but a therapist may be helpful in maximizing abilities and exploring other ways to communicate.

Non-verbal techniques for communicating, such as gesturing or pointing to pictures, may help people express themselves.

Aphasia identification cards explaining that the person has a language problem may be helpful. Many speech pathologists and occupational therapists have their own practices, while others are available through local hospitals and medical centers.

There are no pills yet for PPA. Because of the 30%-40% probability of Alzheimer's disease (AD), some physicians will prescribe AD drugs such as Exelon (rivastigmine), Razadyne (galantamine), Aricept (donepezil) or Namenda (memantine).

None have been shown to improve PPA. Medicine is also sometimes prescribed to manage behavioral symptoms such as depression, anxiety, or agitation, which may occur later in the course of the illness.

There are, however, life-enriching interventions and speech therapies that can help improve a diagnosed person's quality of life.

The primary goal of treatment for language impairments in individuals with PPA is to improve the ability to communicate.

Because the type of language problems experienced by patients with PPA may vary, the focus of treatment for improving communication ability will also vary.

A complete speech and language evaluation provides the information needed to determine the type of treatment that is most appropriate.

There are two basic approaches to speech therapy for PPA.

One approach is to focus treatment directly on the language skills that are impaired (for example, skills to enhance word-retrieval abilities), and the other is to provide augmentative/alternative communication strategies or devices.

The current recommendation is that both treatment approaches be used in people with PPA.

Regardless of which strategies are provided to people with PPA, it is important that the family is involved in treatment and that the use of the strategy in the natural environment is encouraged.

Ernestina Connolly

Chapter 29

How Dan Currently Communicates With the Outside World

As mentioned previously, most aphasic patients develop a set of compensatory verbal skills to indicate their needs and desires.

Here is the communication set that Dan currently utilizes.

Terms that Dan uses to communicate:

Normal – could means several things, he is doing okay nothing hurts, not hungry, or does not want anything to eat or drink

Temporarily – means we will be right back or come back with more Coke (he loves Coke)

Literally – He always starts a sentence with the word literally

As a matter of Fact – He sometimes starts a sentence with these words.

Error/Bad – Throw trash away or food is no longer good; if you bump into Dan, he will say you did an error for me, or if you drop something that belongs to him, he will tell you that it was bad or you did an error

Big Item – Large or I'm full

Person – This could mean many things, dog, or an actual person, place or thing.

Up top – can mean up the street, or up the canyon or rain, sun or clouds

Item – Could mean the dog, car, truck, food, or anything else in the house he cannot remember the name of

Video – could mean camera, computer, TV, or remote control

Order – means he wants to pay the bill or have I ordered something to eat; or he wants to take me out to for dinner

I love the person – could mean he likes the dog or the music or the food he is eating, or mutual friends

I do everything perfect – means he makes no mistakes

Other active skills that Dan has:

Dan knows how to:

- Get to and from home and anywhere in California or Arizona.

- Get to his parent's house in Wildomar, Long Beach and his brother's house;

- Get to my parent's home in Victorville; his daughter's home in Prescott, Arizona.

- Dan does not know the names of Cities he is trying to get to, only North, South, East and West;

He:

- Helps clean the house, washes dishes, does laundry, mows the lawn, fixes many things that need fixing and then shows you what he did;

- Cannot read or write, but can build anything or put anything together just by looking at a picture of what it's supposed to look like;

- Can tell you the date of when he bought a certain item or when we visited a specific place when he was a child or a young adult;

- Cannot tell you the name of the restaurant or food he wants to eat, but he direct you how to get there.

- He knows how to order what he wants by pointing at the item or saying the actual cost of the item on the board, or if there is a picture with a number he will say number 4, only number 4 and a coke.

- He loves hamburgers, Chinese food, Italian food and Subway sandwiches, Top Raman, hot dogs and a nice medium rare steak and baked potatoes.

- If he wants to make you happy, he will play the music you like to listen to; Dan thinks he is the best dancer in the crowd, then when I assure him that he is the best dancer, it puts a smile on his face.

- He loves opening presents and truly appreciates what you give him; he is grateful when you bring him food or take him out to eat and always says thank you very much.

If he wants to take you out to eat, he will say he will order for you and say "I order what you order."

Names or words he is familiar with are:

- Phone, Chicken, Burger, Coke; Mother, Dad, brother Mike, Eric; Erni; Springer; Sportster , ChuChu (our dogs), Margaret, Nicki and Gino;

He:

- Still knows which motorcycle parts go with which bike – Harley Davidson or Triumph

- Still knows how to fix my computer and order products online.

- Orders food by the number displayed on board

- Remembers the cost of an item at a restaurant or the cost of gasoline;

- Knows how to go online and check the balances of our banks accounts and if I borrow money from our savings account, he makes sure I put it back;
- Remembers various email passwords;

- Is very good with money, does not spend more than he has;

- Loves Baskin Robins ice cream and says he wants 31;

If he cannot tell you what he wants, he will show you on the computer or show you how to get to where he wants to go.

For instance, if he wants something to eat, he will direct you as to where he wants to go to get something to eat. He will say make a left, right or points to go straight ahead. He does not do well when you yell at him. You cannot tell him he did something wrong or he did an error, because he does everything perfect;

He:

- Has a daily routine each morning, gets up at 6:00 or 6:30 a.m., feeds the dogs, then he takes the dogs for a 2 mile walk every day, 7 days a week.

- Waters the grass for half an hour in the morning and in the evening

- Feeds the dogs in the evening at 5:00 p.m. If we are out and about, he makes sure we get home in time to feed the dogs.

- Loves his dogs and makes sure they are safe at home

Chapter 30

What Can We Now Expect In Terms of Dan's PPA

Dan may become mute and may eventually lose the ability to understand written or spoken language (Dan currently has difficulty understanding written or spoken language)

His memory may become impaired and may develop other neurological conditions over time and eventually he will need day-to-day care.

People with primary progressive aphasia may also develop behavior or social problems, such as being anxious, irritable or aggressive, poor judgment and inappropriate social behavior.

The aggressiveness has now started to begin with Dan. If Dan wants to do something that maybe dangerous he will do it, like cutting down a wire from the neighbor's house that had fallen to our side of the driveway.

I tried to get Dan to stop pulling the wire down because I didn't know if it was a live wire or not, but he would not listen to me.

When he finally got it down from the neighbor's home, he then got one of the ladders and was going to climb the telephone pole to try and pull the wire down. When I tried to remove the ladder, Dan yelled at me and pushed me and said "you're doing an error."

Dan has never pushed or shoved or even raised his voice to me in the past, so I have to be careful not to get him upset, otherwise, he will throw and break whatever he has in his hands or kick whatever is near to him.   A couple of times he has already swung his right arm out of frustration when I take something away from him.   Thank God I happen to be on the left side of him; otherwise, I would get hit.

I am not afraid for my safety, because I know Dan would never hurt me intentionally.   I just have to make sure I don't take things away from him that are going to get him upset.   Something I definitely have to work on so Dan won't hurt me or hurt himself.

Ernestina Connolly

Chapter 31

Final Thoughts – Closing

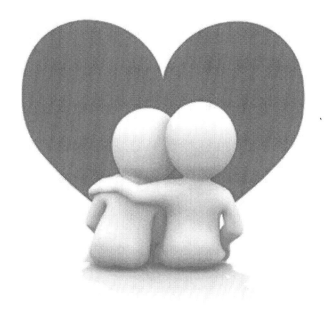

Dan and I are happier now than ever and our communication, although sometimes a difficult process to understand, is getting better. We have our own way of communicating which works for us.

I describe it as having a child who is learning to speak and says certain words in his or her language. Somehow, you pick it up because they say the same thing when they want something or when they are trying to tell you something. When he makes a complete sentence, or says a new word, I get so excited.

If you are around Dan on a daily or weekly basis, you will be able to understand his language and be able to communicate with him. It just takes time and patience to understand what Dan is trying to say.

Dan is still very bright, knows exactly what he wants, and although he's unable to verbally tell you his thoughts, he can guide you to what he is talking about.

Sometimes, he can draw what he is searching for which is pretty amazing considering all that he has gone through and is still going though. He continues to amaze me each day with all the things he can still do. I believe a lot has to do with Dan's photographic memory.

It's the little things in life that make me happy and that make Dan happy too. I love to watch Dan take pictures of everything and anything and then have him show me, on the computer, all the pictures he took.

Sometimes they can be the same picture, but with a different camera, or should I say, with one of the fifty cameras Dan has collected since his was diagnosed with PPA.

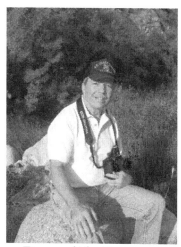

It's not easy caring for a loved one with PPA, but it is rewarding when you see the changes and challenges that they go through and the achievements they

Dan with Camera

accomplish on a daily, weekly or monthly basis.

Finally, I want to thank God for giving me the serenity, potency, valor, and the knowledge to understand Dan's condition, and for making this whole state of affairs a positive experience.

I also want to express gratitude to my entire family and friends for their unrelenting love, support, their kindness, and for providing me the strength to get through this intricate time of our lives (I can't name everyone, but you know who you are).

I'm especially grateful to my family at AGC, who supported me as well, allowing me the time off to adjust my work schedule so I could spend more time with Dan, and for getting me through the tough times.

Honestly, I couldn't have done it without all of you because we all need support from someone.
It's difficult, challenging, and scary to face these kinds of crises alone, so don't be afraid to solicit aid because that is what families and friends are for.

I am truly blessed to have a magnificent husband who didn't give up on us, and who still has the fortitude to put up with me.

I am proud of myself for taking action, for both my husband as well as myself, so we could push onward and continue to be strong.

"DECISIONS YOU MAKE DICTATE YOUR FUTURE"

By Ernestina Connolly

Our Wedding Vows

> ### Our wedding vows and the commitment we made to one another ring true.
>
> "Daniel, I promise you my love today, and always without limit;
>
> To always be near you when we are apart; to take care of you and support you. You are my best friend, my soul-mate, my love and my life. I will respect you as my husband and my Sweetiepie. I promise to love you for as long as we both shall live."
>
> "Ernestina, I want to share my life with you; I promise to protect you and be by your side. I want to explore the world with you, and to create a home with you. I'm committed to our future together. I will respect you as my wife and my Sweetiepie. I promise to love you for as long as we both shall live."
>
> 10/13/06

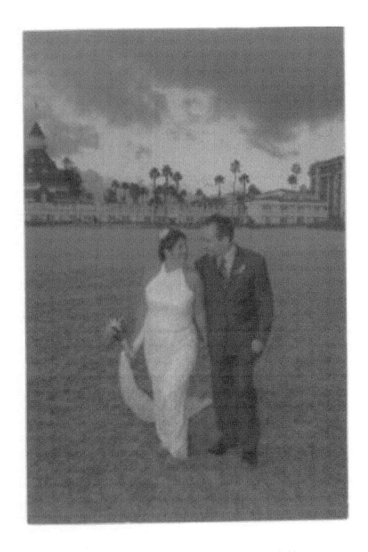

Ernestina and Dan - Our wedding

October 13, 2006

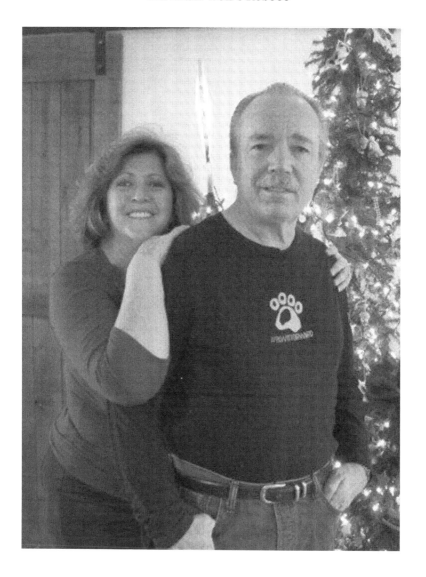

Erni & Dan – Xmas 2014

Epilogue

This book has been written as our story has unfolded and it will never really be finished until Dan is gone.

Even though Dan's communication is limited now, I still understand what he is saying or trying to tell me. It's been a work in progress since February 10, 2012, when Dan became disabled and was unable to work.

Dan is also so much happier now and I can see it in his touch and expressions.

We make each other happy all the time.

Life is simple, and even though it is complicated sometimes, we appreciate one another now more than ever and everyone around me can see it too.

Life is good.

Made in the USA
Lexington, KY
25 July 2015